Atlas of OCT

NOTICE: The OCT Atlas is not intended as a diagnostic guide and is not a substitute for clinical experience and judgment. When diagnosing and treating patients, each clinician must analyze and interpret all available data and make individual clinical decisions based on his or her clinical judgment and experience.

Table of Contents

The Normal Retina 1

Posterior Vitreous Detachments 6

Vitreomacular Traction 8

Epiretinal Membrane 11

Lamellar Macular Hole 14

Full Thickness Macular Hole 16

Cystoid Macular Edema 17

Cysts, Exudates, and Outer Retinal Holes 19

Diabetic Macular Edema 20

Dry Macular Degeneration 21

Wet Macular Degeneration 25

Central Serous Chorioretinopathy 30

Multiple Pathologies 31

The Normal Retina

The first step in interpreting optical coherence tomography (OCT) images is understanding the layers of the retina as observed in a "normal" retina, or a retina without macular pathology.

The image below is an enlargement of a cross sectional image of a "normal" retina obtained from a spectral domain OCT. The right half of the figure is the actual image obtained from the OCT. The left half of the figure is a gray-scale enhancement of the image. Also, the margins of the retinal layers have been artificially enhanced in the left half of the figure, to enable readers to better identify the retinal layers.

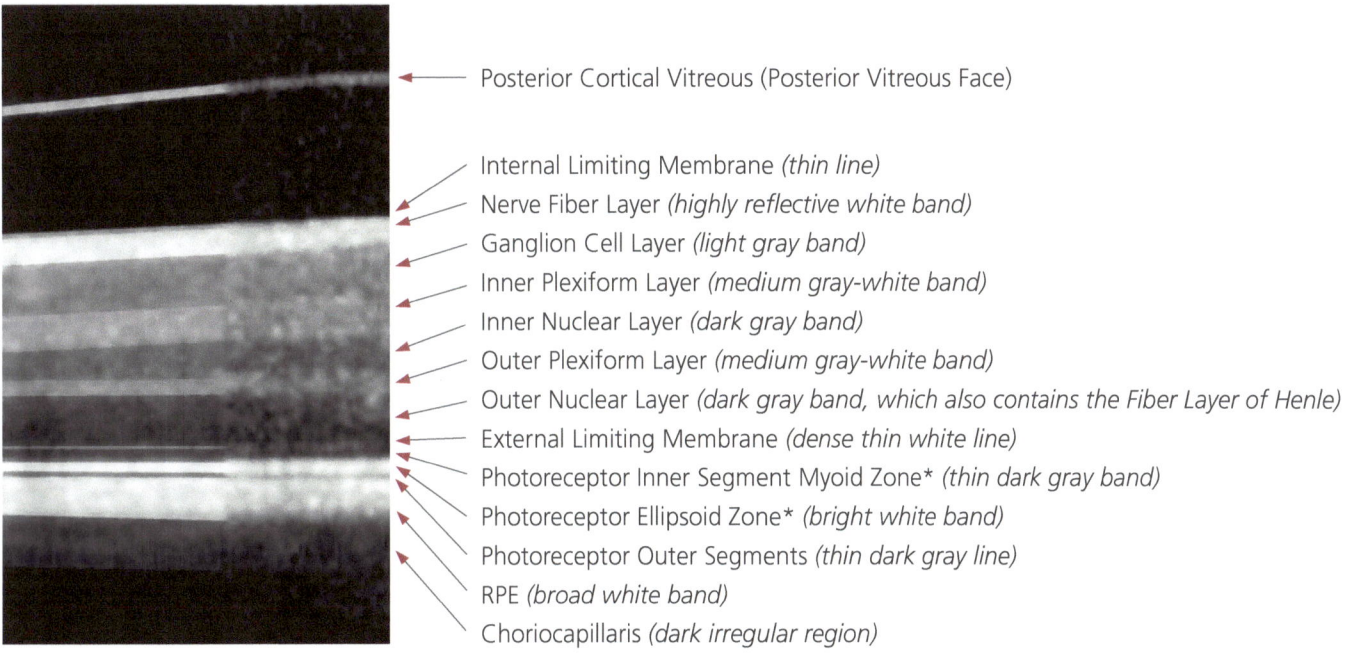

- Posterior Cortical Vitreous (Posterior Vitreous Face)
- Internal Limiting Membrane *(thin line)*
- Nerve Fiber Layer *(highly reflective white band)*
- Ganglion Cell Layer *(light gray band)*
- Inner Plexiform Layer *(medium gray-white band)*
- Inner Nuclear Layer *(dark gray band)*
- Outer Plexiform Layer *(medium gray-white band)*
- Outer Nuclear Layer *(dark gray band, which also contains the Fiber Layer of Henle)*
- External Limiting Membrane *(dense thin white line)*
- Photoreceptor Inner Segment Myoid Zone* *(thin dark gray band)*
- Photoreceptor Ellipsoid Zone* *(bright white band)*
- Photoreceptor Outer Segments *(thin dark gray line)*
- RPE *(broad white band)*
- Choriocapillaris *(dark irregular region)*

The labeled cross section above may be used to identify the layers in the "normal" retina below. The image is a horizontal cross-section through the fovea.

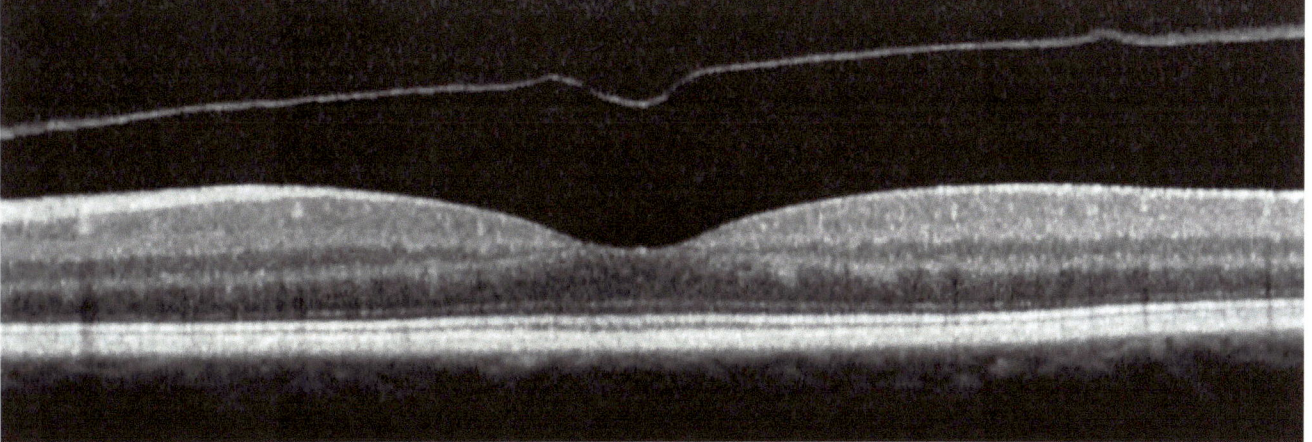

The Photoreceptor Ellipsoid Zone is the portion of the inner segment of the photoreceptors, that is immediately adjacent to the junction between photoreceptor inner and outer segments. This "ellipsoid zone" of the inner segments is packed with mitochondria. The recent International Nomenclature for OCT Panel has proposed that this hyperreflective layer be referred to as the "ellipsoid zone" rather than what has been previously believed to be the junction between the inner and outer segments of photoreceptors. While there is not yet definitive evidence to determine this hyperreflective layer's actual anatomical correlate, and though there is controversy in nomenclature, for the purposes of this atlas, the "consensus" term "ellipsoid zone" shall be adopted until further data is available.

The Photoreceptor Inner Segment Myoid Zone is the portion of the inner segment of photoreceptors that is between the mitocondria-rich ellipsoid zone and the cell body / nucleus of the photoreceptor inner segments. This myoid zone is rich in protein synthesis apparatus, which results in poor reflectivity on the OCT.

The Normal Retina

Retinal Layers and Cell Types

In the first image below, the superimposed illustration is a representational drawing of the cell types found in a normal fovea (cells not to scale). In the second image, the representational drawing is color coded by cell type.

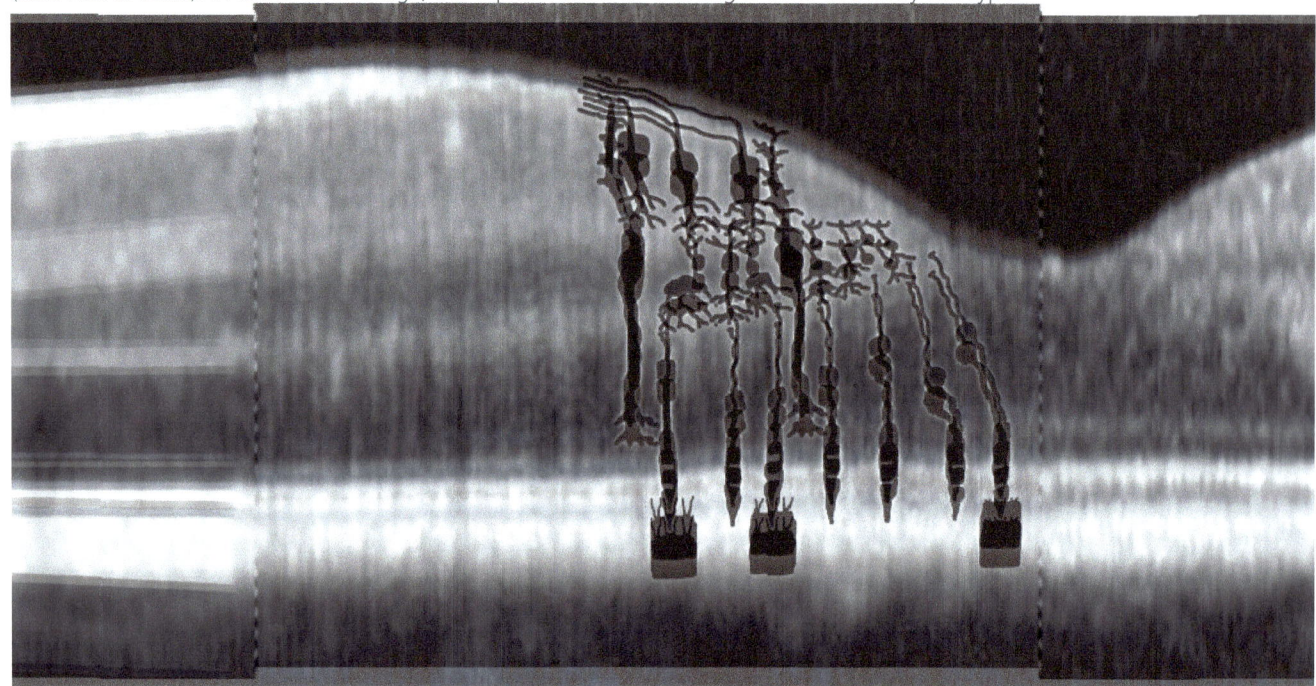

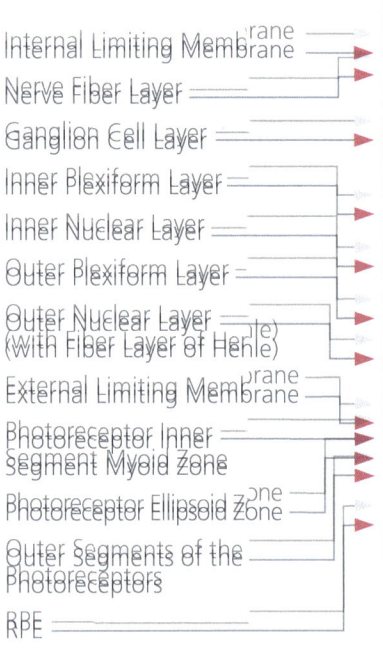

Internal Limiting Membrane
Nerve Fiber Layer
Ganglion Cell Layer
Inner Plexiform Layer
Inner Nuclear Layer
Outer Plexiform Layer
Outer Nuclear Layer (with Fiber Layer of Henle)
External Limiting Membrane
Photoreceptor Inner Segment Myoid Zone
Photoreceptor Ellipsoid Zone
Outer Segments of the Photoreceptors
RPE

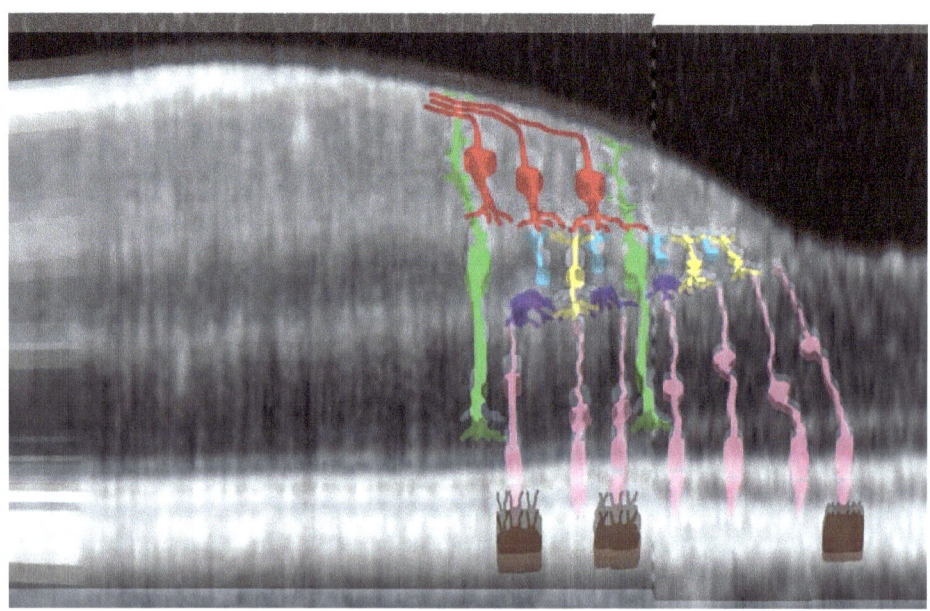

Ganglion Cells
Bipolar Neurons
Horizontal Neurons
RPE

Müller Glial Cells
Amacrine Neurons
Photoreceptors

The Normal Retina

Outer Retinal Layers

In this scan of a healthy retina, notice that the most hyper-reflective (brightest white) band is composed of more than one line. It is a common misconception that this band is composed solely of retinal pigment epithelium (RPE). The detailed images produced by the SPECTRALIS system have shown that this band is composed of two distinct major bands (the ellipsoid zone of the photoreceptors and the RPE). In the second image, the line highlighted in red is the ellipsoid zone of the photoreceptors. The band highlighted in green is the RPE; this band often appears as two close but separate lines.

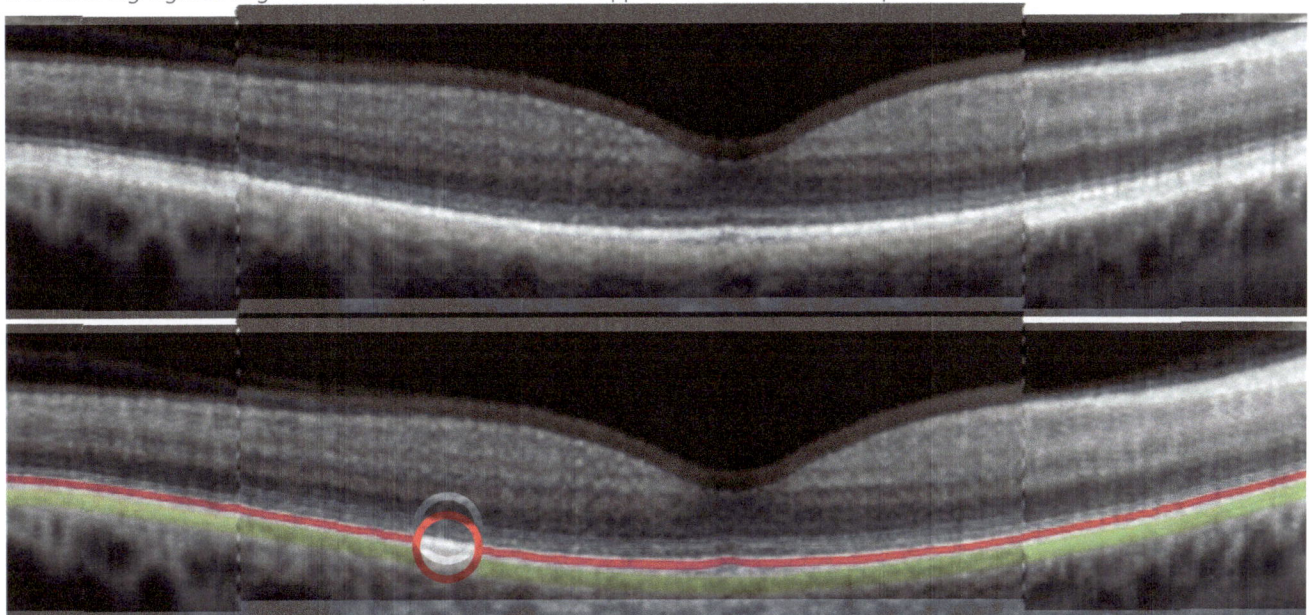

In many SPECTRALIS images, the RPE layer (highlighted in green in the image above) is seen to consist of two distinct white layers. One of these (highlighted in yellow in the image at right) is believed to be the inner membrane of the RPE cells, which is adjacent to the photoreceptors. The other layer within the RPE band (highlighted in blue in the image at right) is believed to be the outer membrane of the RPE cells. Along with Bruch's membrane this tissue forms part of the RPE cells' basement membrane. This outer membrane of the RPE is adjacent to the choriocapillaris and choroid.

The two lines of the RPE are believed to be a result of elongations in the inner membrane of the RPE cells adjacent to the photoreceptors. The inner membrane of the RPE cells forms elongated contact cylinders that wrap around, or interdigitate with, the outer segments of cones located outside the fovea (labeled 1 in the image to the right). The cones within the fovea have contact cylinders that are less elongated, and the inner membranes remain closer to the RPE cell bodies (labeled 2 in the image to the right). The inner membranes do not wrap substantially around rods; therefore, outside the fovea, a portion of the inner membranes is further away from the outer membrane of the RPE cells; it is in this perifoveal region that the RPE sometimes appears as two distinct bands. While the inner-most of these two distinct bands (yellow in image at right) is sometimes referred to the Interdigitation Zone, it is believed to be more a feature of the distance between the outer and inner-most membranes of the RPE cells than the interdigitations. These lines, whether single or double, should not be confused for the ellipsoid zone of the photoreceptors.

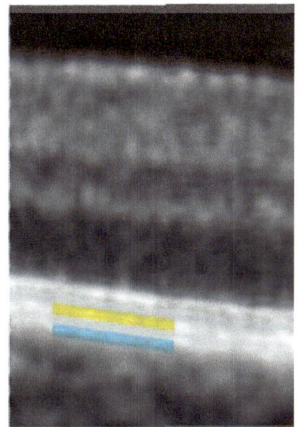

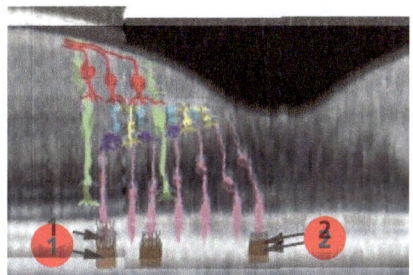

The Normal Retina

Photoreceptors & Vitreous

The outer segments of the photoreceptors appear as a dark band that is located between the RPE (highlighted in green in the image below) and the ellipsoid zone of the photoreceptors (highlighted in red in the image). The photoreceptors span the entire length between the RPE and the outer plexiform layer and have been shaded orange in the image below.

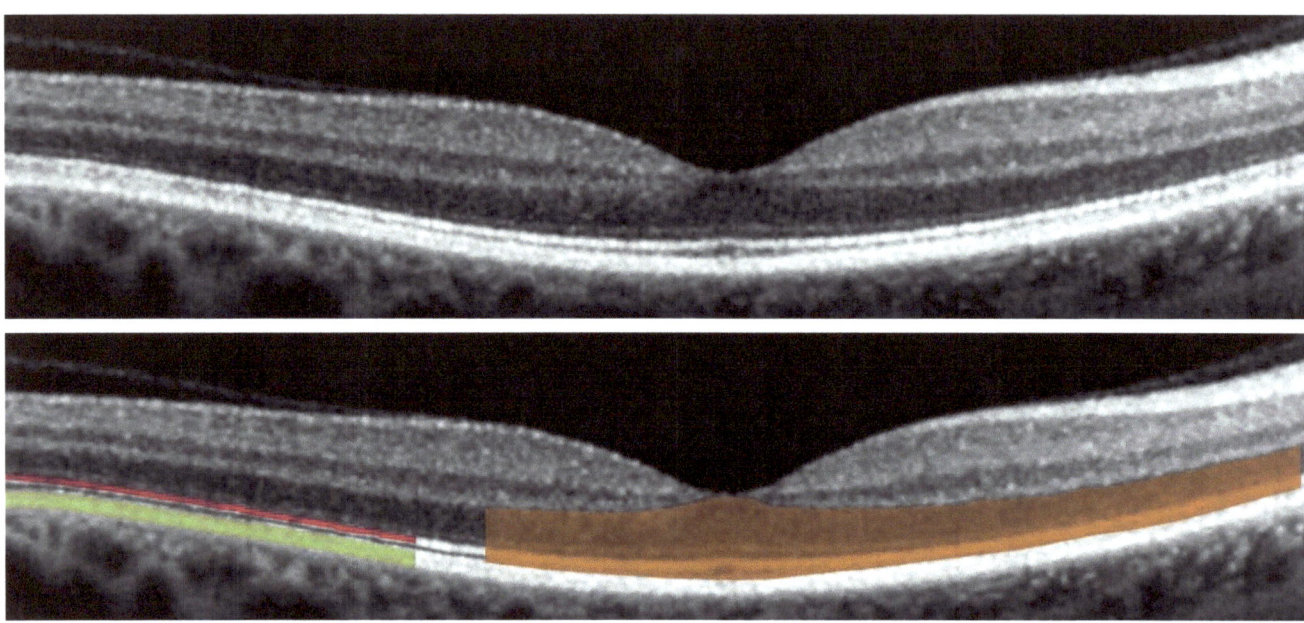

Within the fovea, the outer segments of the photoreceptors are thinner and longer, and so the outer segment band (highlighted in orange in the image above) is thicker. Note how it appears to form a peak (arrowhead in the figure on the right). There are also a greater number of photoreceptor nuclei within the fovea, so the outer nuclear layer, which represents the photoreceptor nuclei, is also thicker within the fovea (indicated by the double-headed arrow in the image to the right).

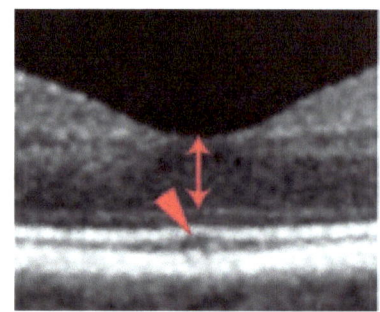

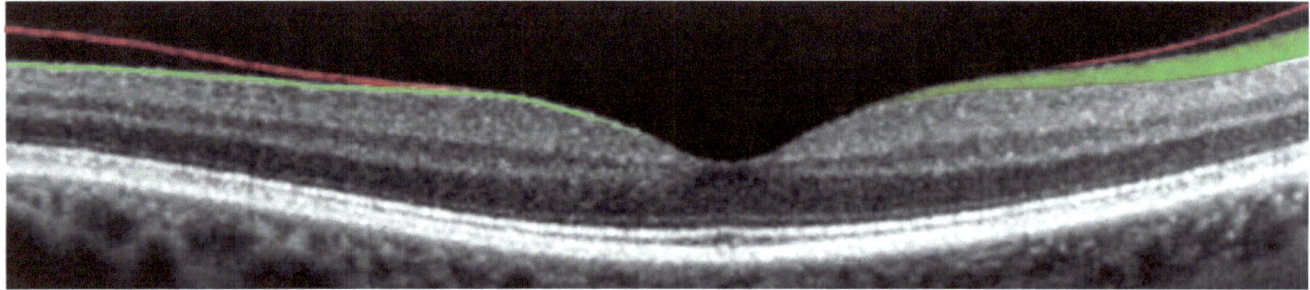

In the image above, the nasal side is easily recognized, because the retinal nerve fiber layer (RNFL) which is highlighted in green, is much thicker nasal to the macula and thinner temporally. The posterior cortical vitreous (shaded red in the image above) attaches to the retina just temporal to the fovea. Clinically, there is no posterior vitreous detachment in this patient, though OCT shows some separation of the posterior vitreous in the temporal and nasal macula and no posterior vitreous detachment through the central macula.

The Normal Retina

Shadows in the Retina

Shadows are created in OCT images by structures or substances that block the transmission of the OCT beam. The dark vertical bands (indicated by the arrows in the image below) are examples of this shadowing effect. In the image below, a venule (red arrowhead) casts a shadow (red arrow), two small arterial capillaries (green arrowheads) cast shadows (green arrows), and a vitreous floater (yellow arrowhead) casts a larger shadow (yellow arrow). The venules and arterial capillaries were determined as such based on fluorescein angiography; this differentiation cannot be made solely on the basis of the information in the OCT scan.

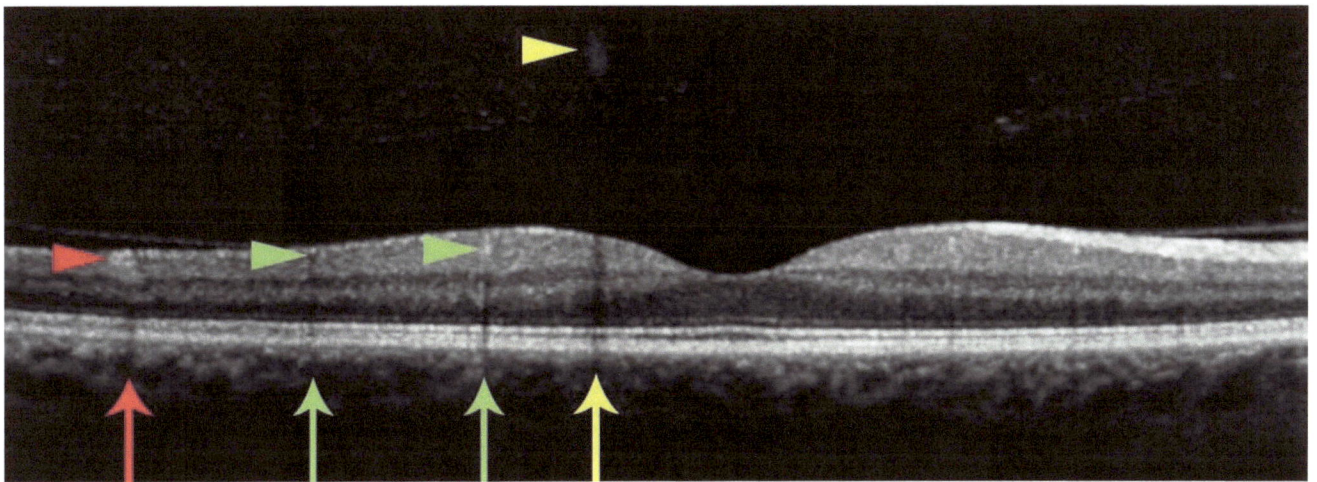

Posterior Vitreous Detachments

The posterior cortical vitreous is often visible on the OCT scan. The information in these scans can assist in determining whether a posterior vitreous detachment (PVD) is present and whether the PVD is complete or incomplete. The images below show a partial PVD. The posterior cortical vitreous (shaded red in the second image) is attached to the nasal retina (arrowhead), but is detached temporally (arrow). Note the numerous vitreous floaters (circle).

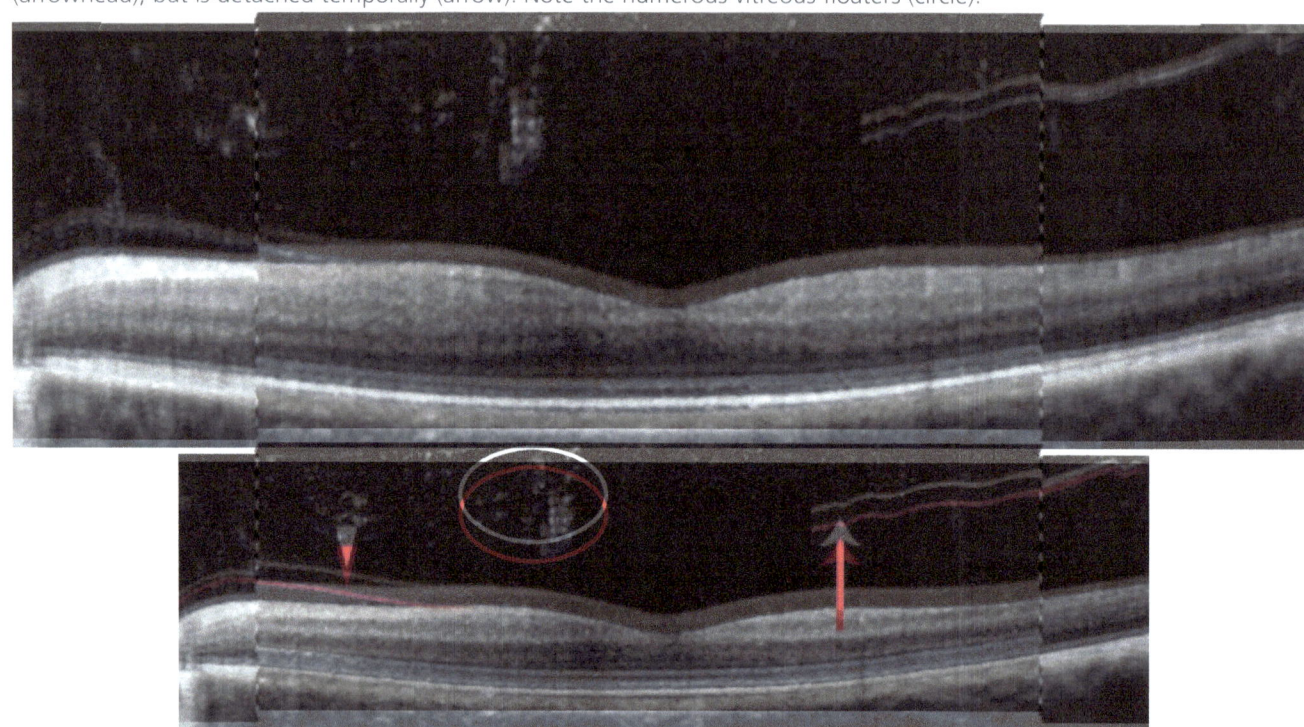

The image below shows a complete PVD. The posterior cortical vitreous (shaded red in the second image) is completely separated from the retina.

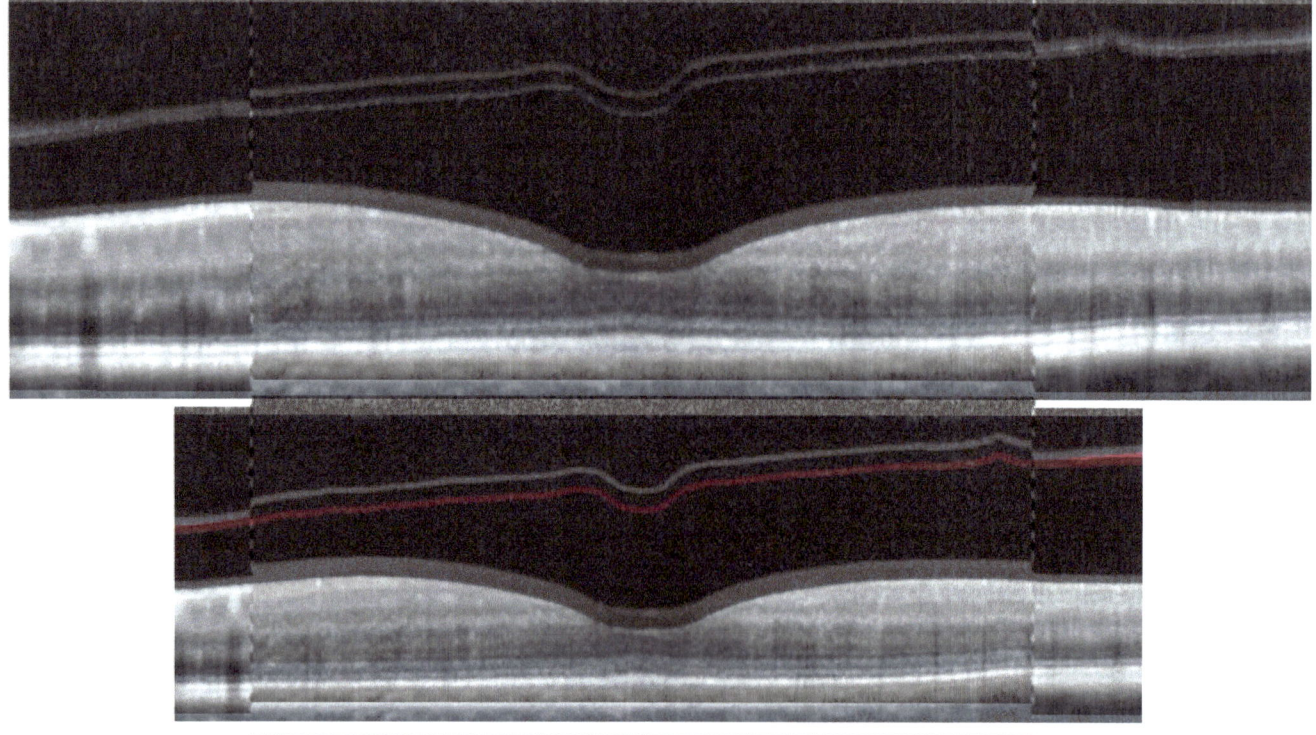

Posterior Vitreous Detachments

PVDs: Early, Complete

The patient below has an early but complete PVD. The mild haziness and graininess of the image is the result of a moderate nuclear sclerotic cataract. Notice that the posterior cortical vitreous (highlighted in red) is very close to the retina in some areas, particularly temporal to the fovea. The bottom set of images capture a section of the retina adjacent to the fovea and clearly demonstrate that the posterior cortical vitreous is separated from the retina.

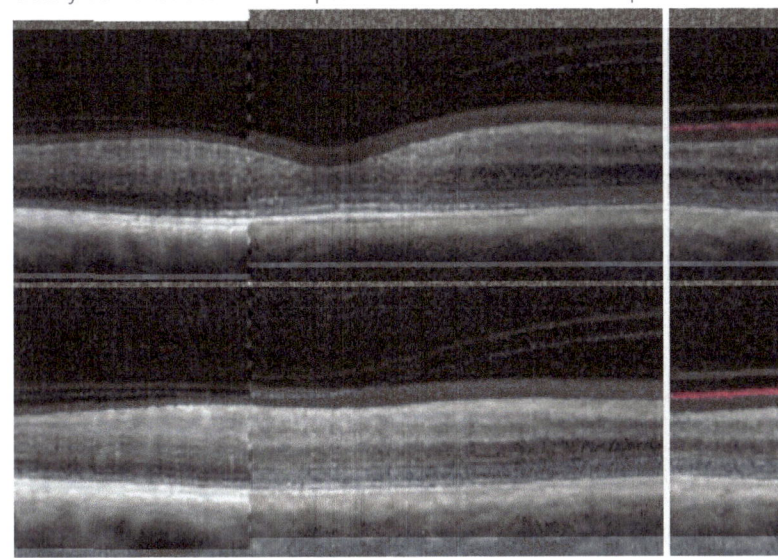
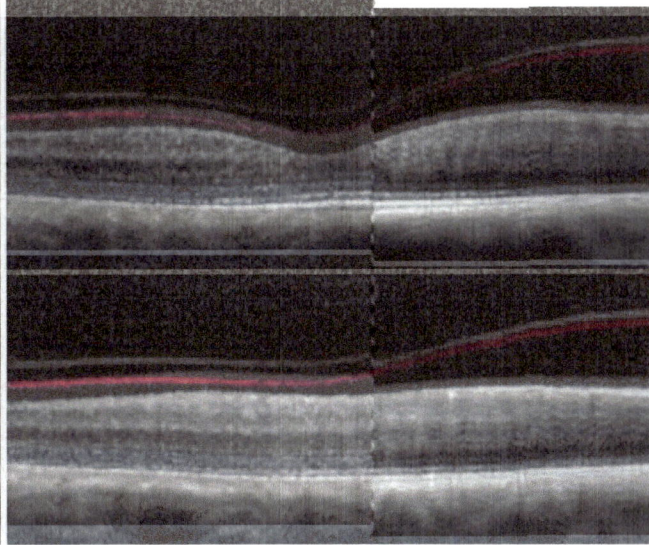

The image below, which is a small section of the image on page 6, shows that the posterior cortical vitreous has an indentation (arrows) that matches the foveal depression. The dense white "spot" within the foveal depression (arrowhead) is not pathologic; it is a specular reflection of the densely reflective outer plexiform layer (the fiber layer of Henle) when it is perpendicular to the light source coming into the eye (shaded green) within the fovea. This white "spot" is not always seen, and its absence does not imply pathology.

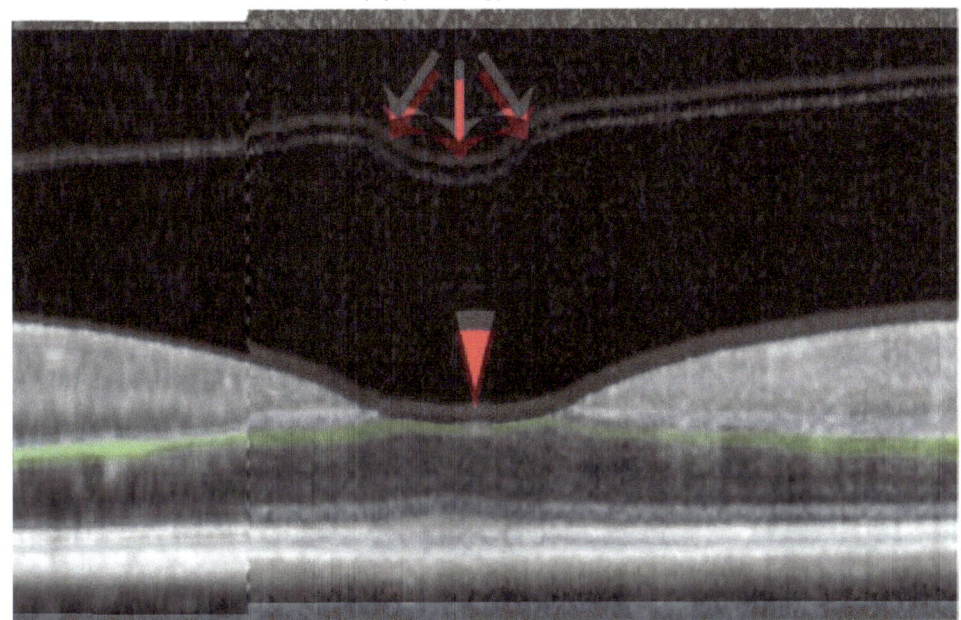

Vitreomacular Traction

The vitreous is densely adherent to the central macula. During vitreous syneresis, the vitreous condenses, which eventually leads to a PVD. However, if the vitreous condenses but does not detach from the central macula, the vitreous will pull on the macula, causing vitreomacular traction (VMT). In the image below, the posterior cortical vitreous (shaded green) is pulling on the fovea, resulting in a peaked appearance (circle) of the ellipsoid zone of the photoreceptors (shaded red).

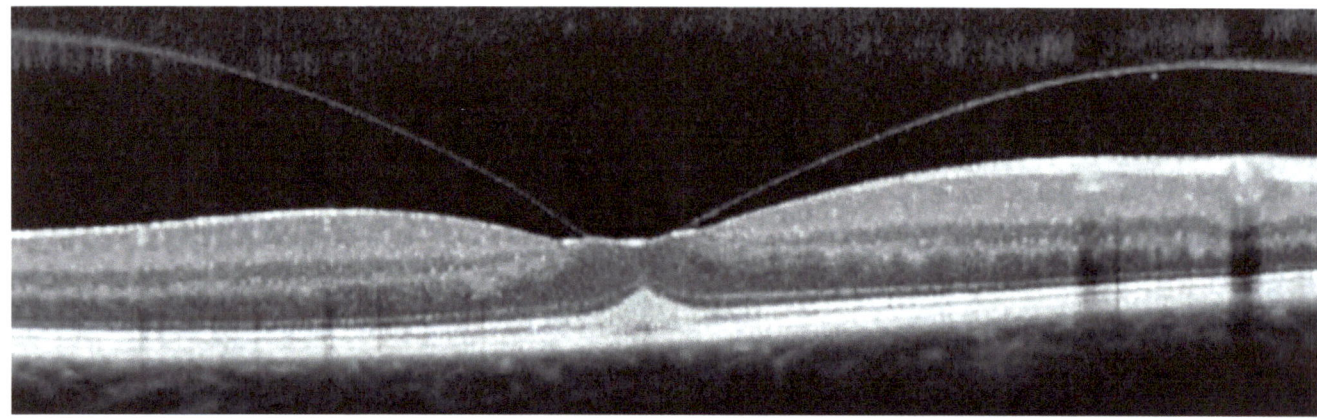

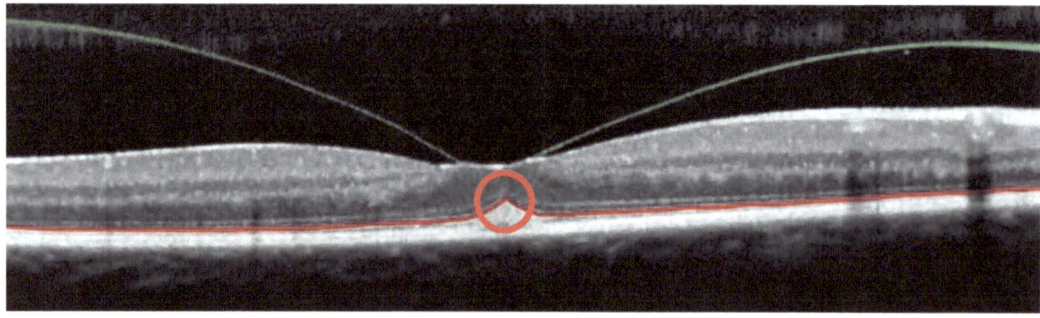

In the VMT case shown below, the pulling from the posterior cortical vitreous (highlighted green) causes retinal thickening and results in retinal distortion (arrow) and intraretinal cyst formation (shaded orange).

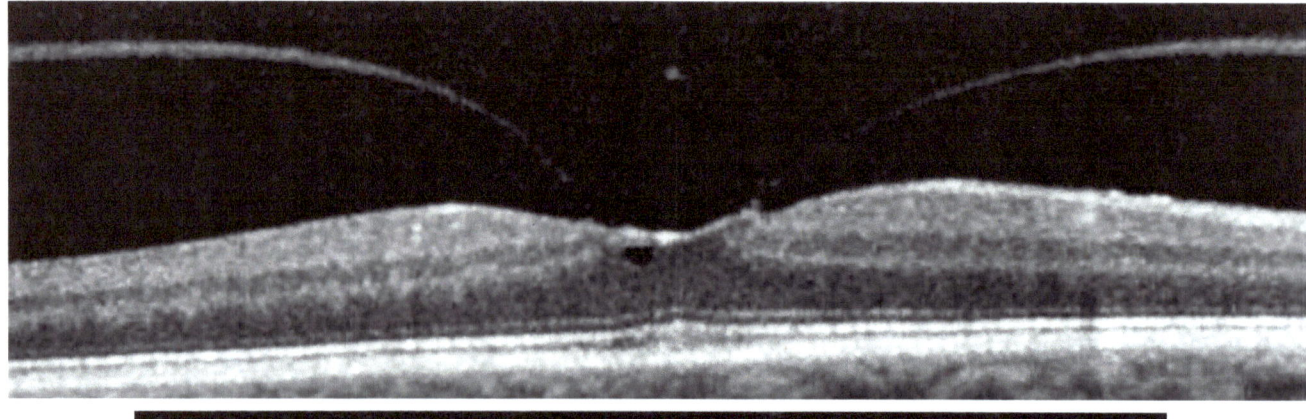

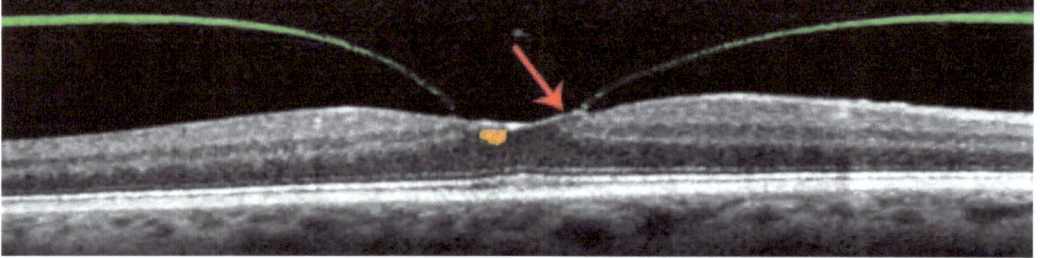

Vitreomacular Traction

VMT: Foveal Cysts

As the posterior cortical vitreous (highlighted red in the image at right below) pulls on the macula, distortion of the retinal architecture can occur, and intraretinal cysts (shaded orange) can develop within the macula. This cystoid macular edema may decrease visual acuity.

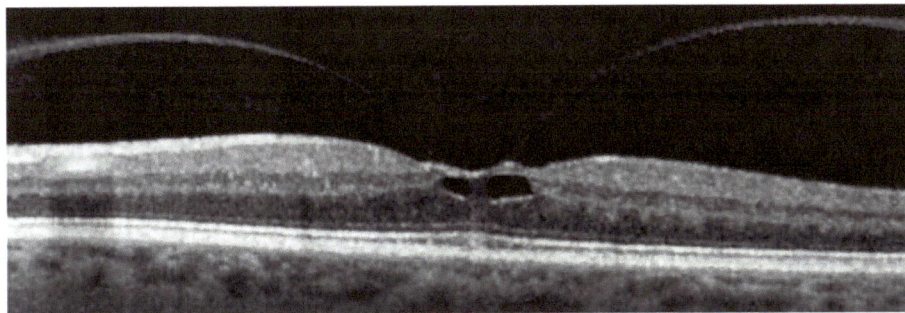
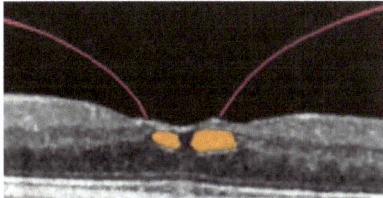

In the image below, the traction from the posterior cortical vitreous (shaded red) is quite extensive. Cystic spaces within the retina (shaded orange) and subretinal fluid (shaded dark blue) are clearly visible. The cystic spaces are open (red arrow) to the vitreous cavity creating a lamellar hole with a roof of retina attached (shaded purple).

The subretinal fluid is located between the retinal pigment epithelium (light blue) and the photoreceptor band. The photoreceptor band is identified by tracing the external limiting membrane (highlighted green), which separates the photoreceptor nuclei from their inner segment myoid zone. Note that the ellipsoid zone of the photoreceptors (highlighted yellow) is only partially visible in this case.

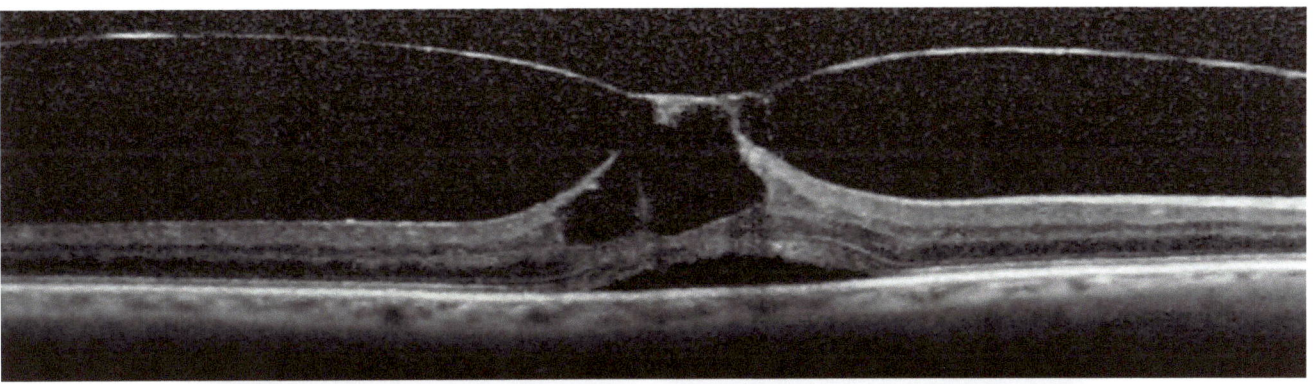
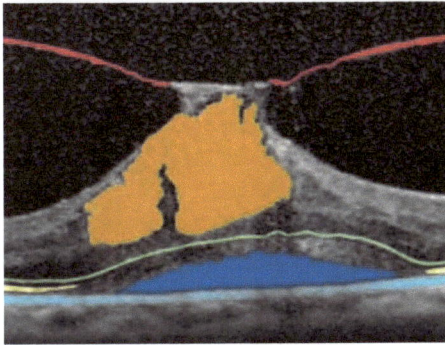
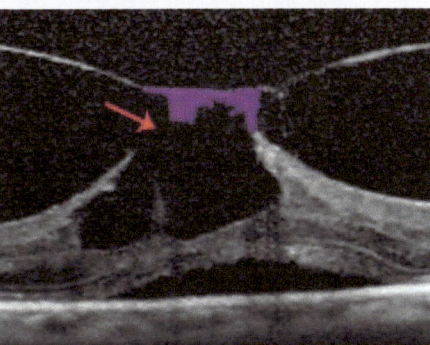

Vitreomacular Traction

VMT: Cysts and Retinal Thickening

In the images below, the traction caused by the posterior cortical vitreous (shaded red), which is still attached to the retina, nasal to the fovea (arrowhead), has resulted in cystoid macular edema (CME). Notice that the intraretinal cysts (shaded orange) are predominantly within the photoreceptor layers. The outer plexiform layer (shaded green) runs above the cysts. This finding is more clearly visible in an adjacent OCT section in the image below to the right. Also, the central cyst has opened to the vitreous cavity, creating a lamellar macular hole (arrow). Retinal structures remain between the lamellar hole and the RPE (shaded yellow):

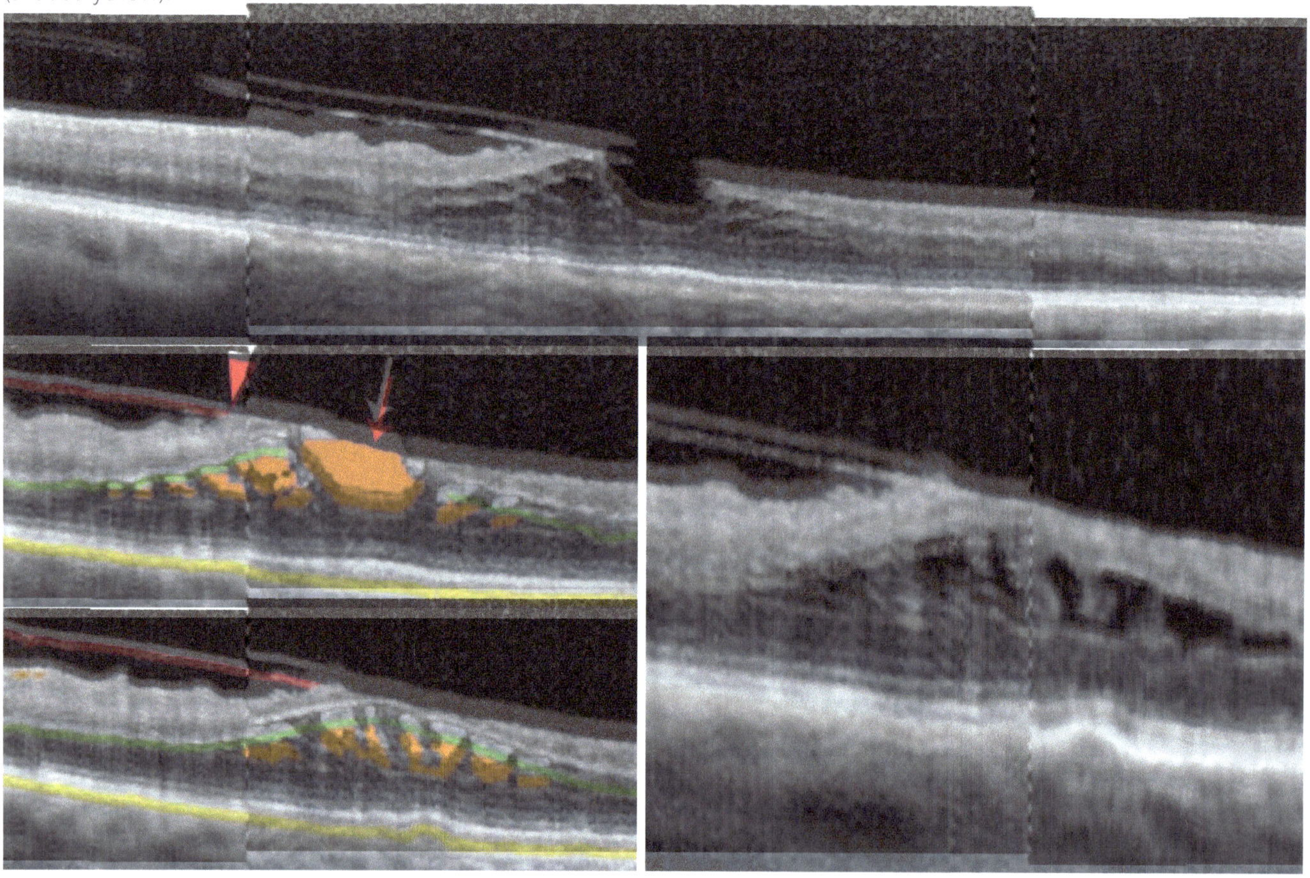

The images below demonstrate a case of VMT through the fovea. The traction from the posterior cortical vitreous (shaded red) causes severe retinal thickening (double-headed arrows):

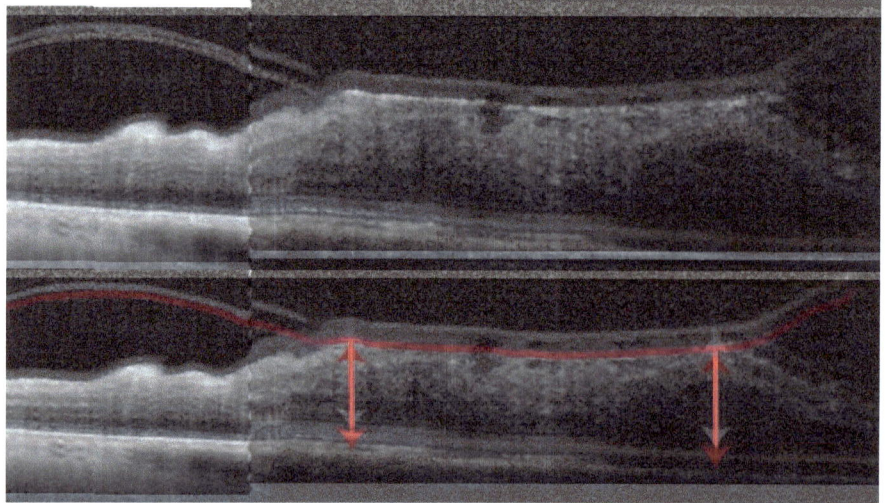

Epiretinal Membrane

In the OCT image below, an epiretinal membrane (shaded red) is attached to the retina in some areas (arrow) and separated in others (arrowhead). The RNFL (shaded green) is often as bright as the epiretinal membrane (ERM), but should not be confused with the ERM. The wrinkling of the retina, seen clinically in the fundus photograph to the bottom right often correlates with undulations within the retina on the OCT. The green line in the fundus photograph represents the location where the OCT scan was obtained.

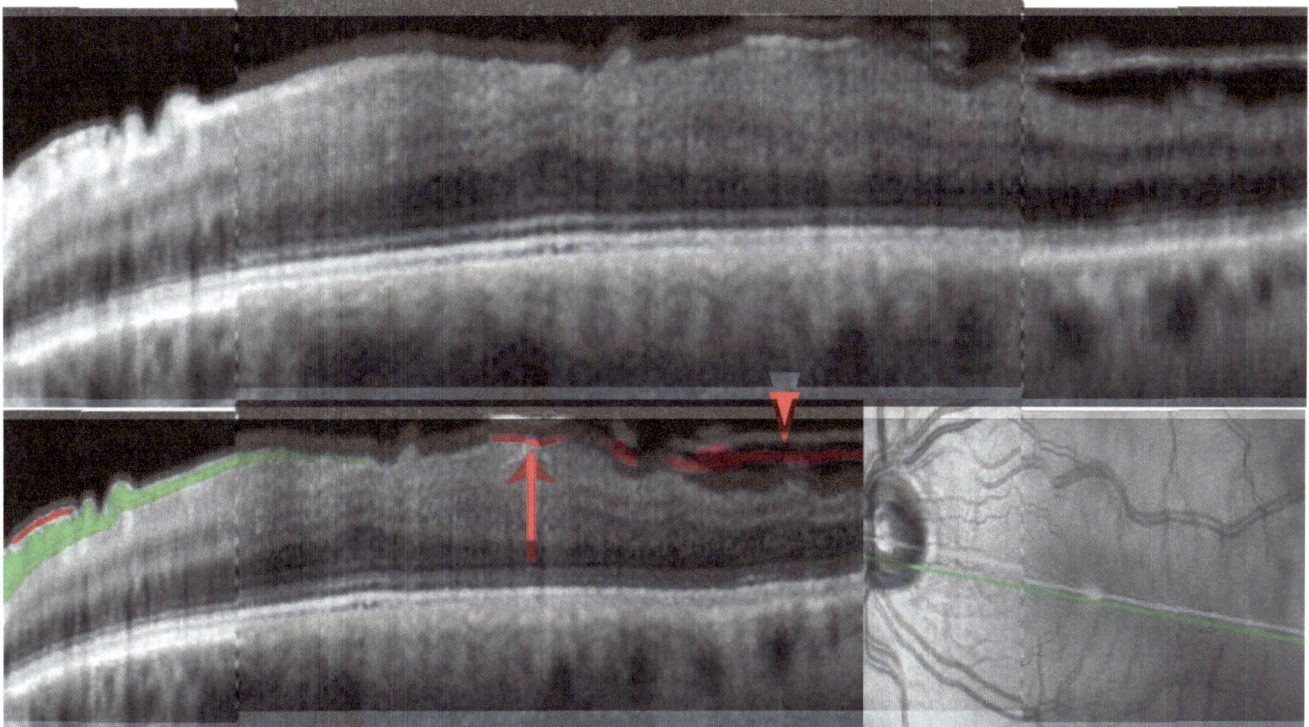

The case below reveals a focal density to the ERM (shaded red with arrow). Again, notice foci of adhesion (arrowheads) of the ERM to the retina. In the corresponding fundus photograph to the bottom right, the green line represents the section through which the OCT scan was obtained. In the superior macula (right most portion of the OCT image), the thickened retina caused by the ERM gradually thins, and the ERM likely extends beyond the area identified by the shaded red line:

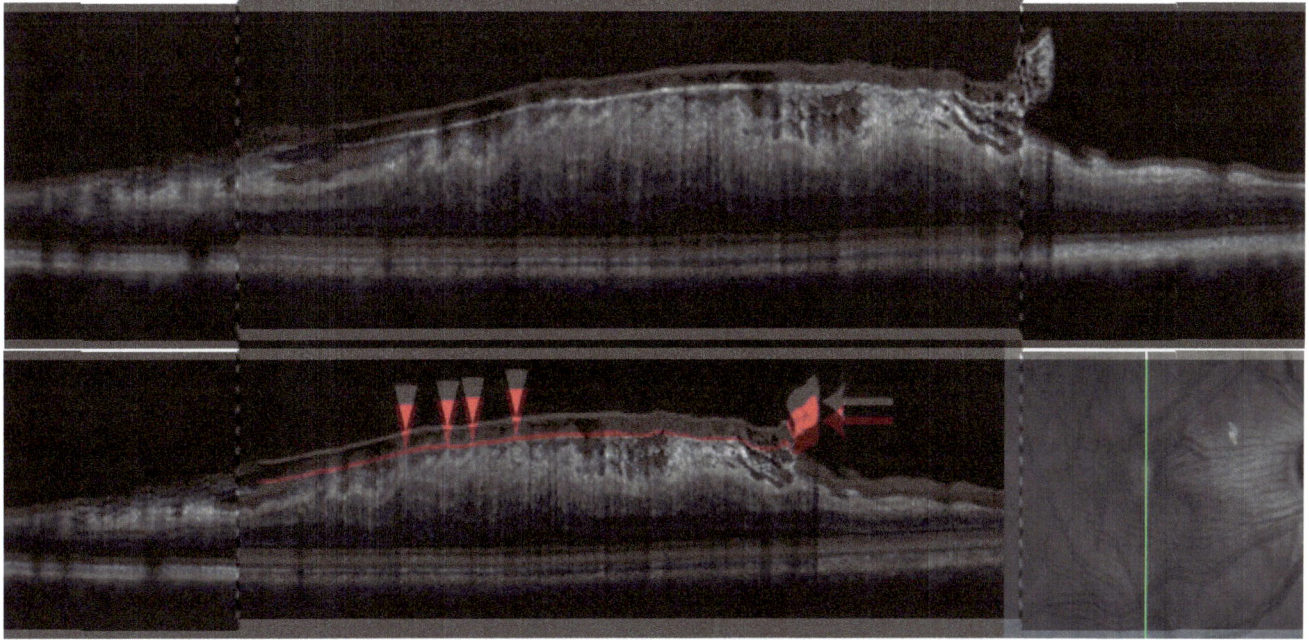

Epiretinal Membrane

ERM: Retinal Distortion

Below, in the OCT image of a patient complaining of visual distortions (metamorphopsias) and blurred vision, the ERM (shaded red) has created traction on the retina. Sometimes it is difficult to distinguish ERM from RNFL in the OCT image, but clinical correlation is often useful in distinguishing between the two. In this section adjacent to the fovea (represented by the central green line in the fundus photograph to the bottom right), the inner nuclear layer (shaded green) has been pulled upwards. Notice the peak (arrow) in the outer nuclear layer.

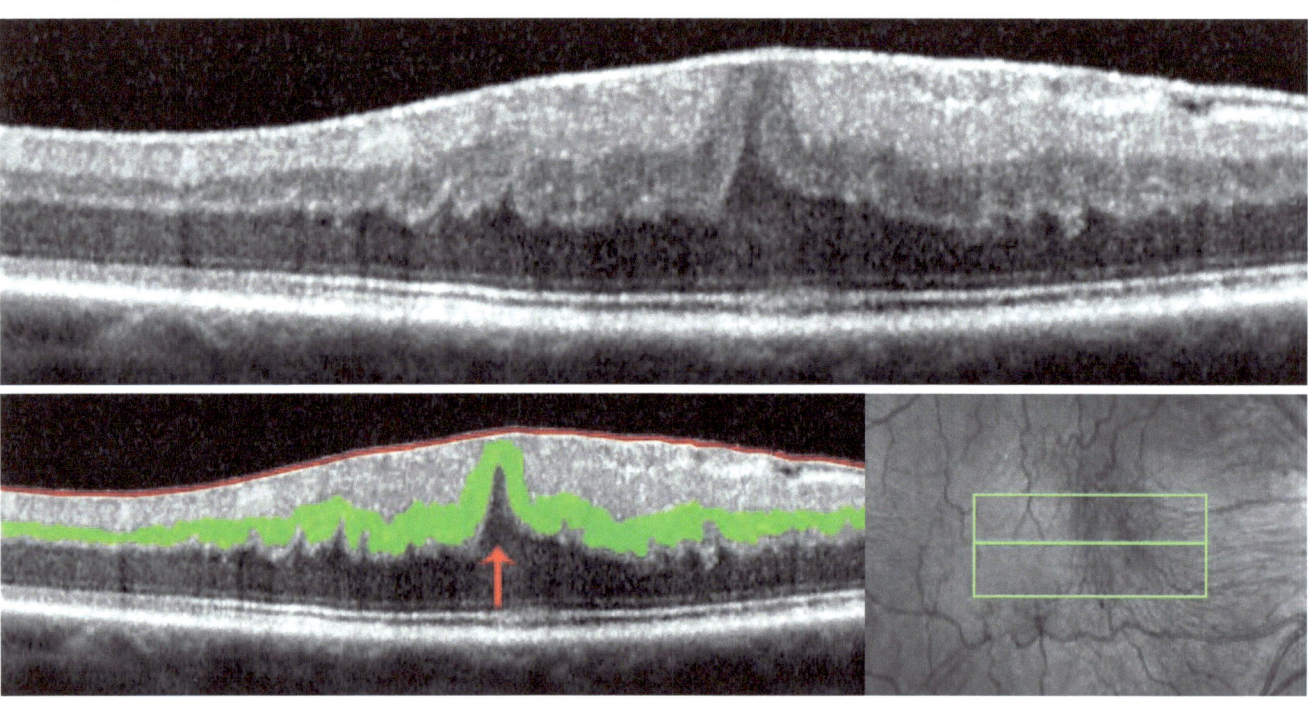

In the case below, the ERM (shaded red) is clinically quite dense, though only portions of it are clearly identifiable on the OCT image. It is tightly adherent to the retina without visible areas of separation. There is also substantial thickening of the retina and the outer nuclear layer (shaded green), representing the photoreceptor nuclei.

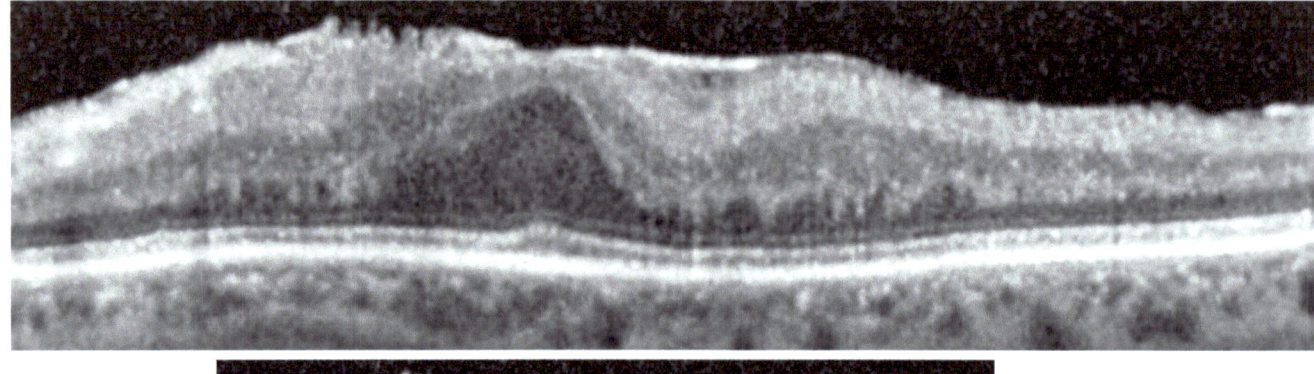

Epiretinal Membrane

ERM: with Lamellar Macular Hole

The traction from the ERM (shaded red) below has resulted in macular edema. There are intraretinal cysts (shaded orange) within the outer nuclear layer and within the inner nuclear layer. Take care not to mistake the RNFL (shaded green) with the ERM, though they often have a similar brightness.

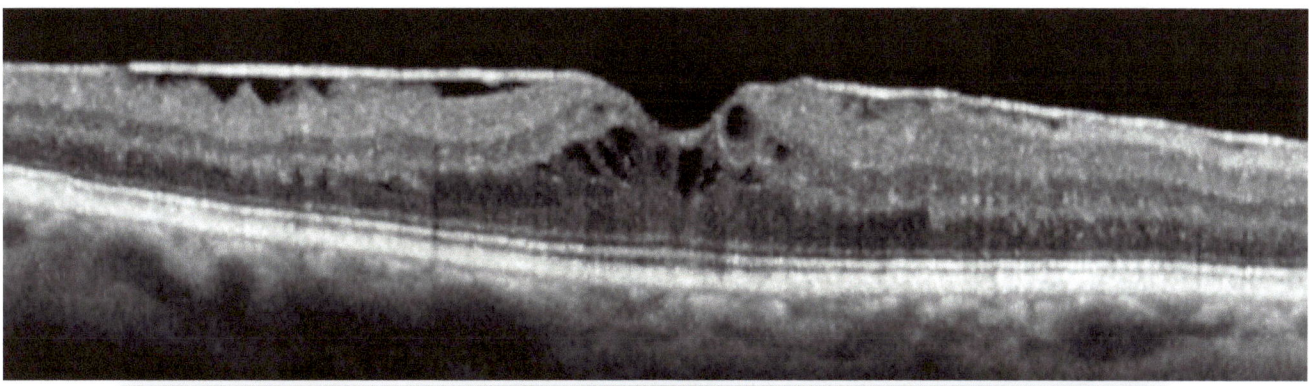

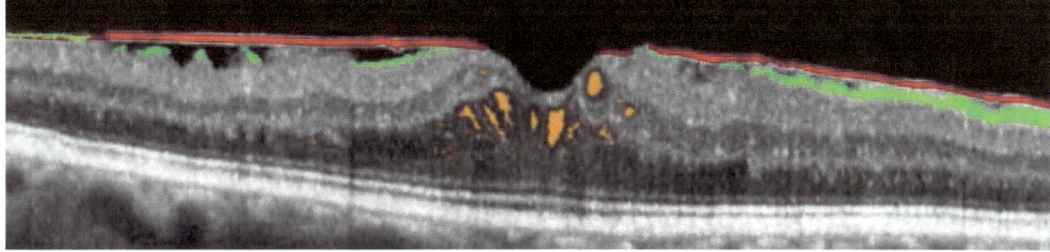

In the OCT image below, the traction from the ERM (shaded red) has also resulted in macular edema, with intraretinal cysts (shaded orange) within the outer nuclear layer. In addition, a lamellar macular hole (arrow) has formed, likely as a result of an opening of an intraretinal cyst and/or traction from the ERM. This patient had 20/20 vision in this eye. The photoreceptor band within the foveola (arrow), particularly the inner and outer segments, demonstrates relatively normal architecture on the OCT. As with the image above, the ERM has areas of close opposition to the retina and areas of separation from the retina.

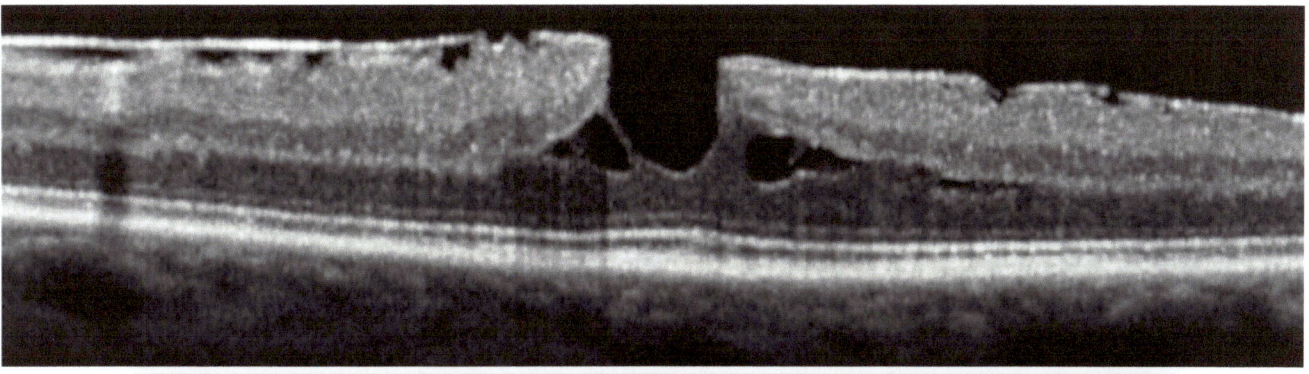

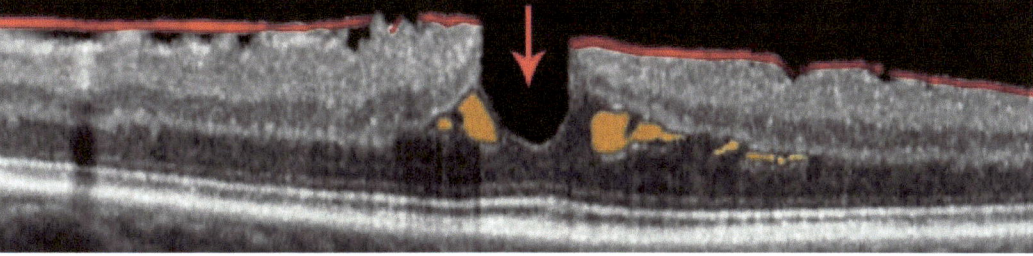

Lamellar Macular Hole

Lamellar macular holes come in many different shapes and extents. Frequently, they can arise from VMT and/or CME, as observed in the image at the bottom of page 9. Other cases arise from an ERM, as observed on page 13. Below are two cases of subtle lamellar macular holes. In the image below, the lamellar macular hole is very small (arrow). While the hole is open to the vitreous cavity, the RPE remains covered by retinal tissue.

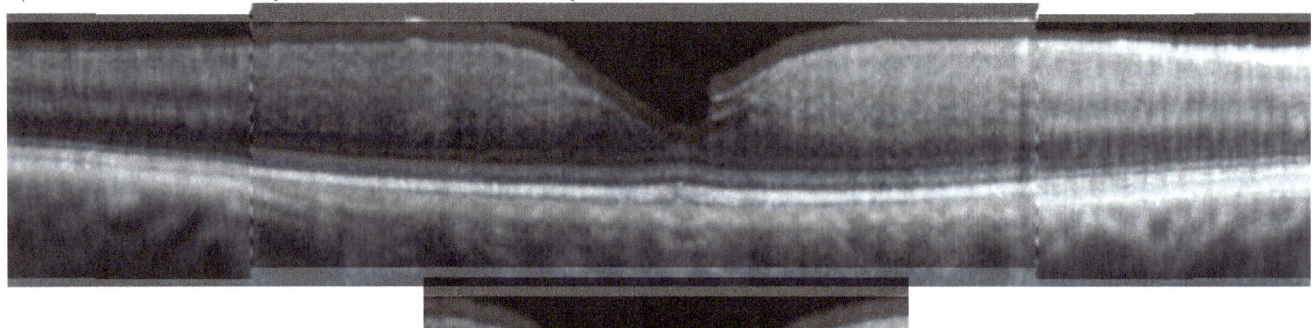

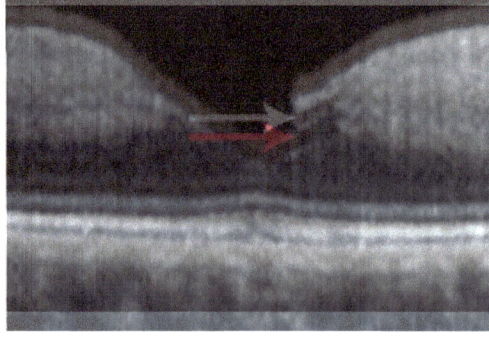

In the case below, the large lamellar macular hole may look similar to a full thickness macular hole because of the upward curling of the inner retinal layers. However, notice that the hole does not go all the way through the retinal layers and appears to stop at the boundary of the outer nuclear layer (shaded green). An ERM (red line) and intraretinal cysts (shaded orange) are also visible. On the right side of the image, the ERM is causing the RNFL to thicken.

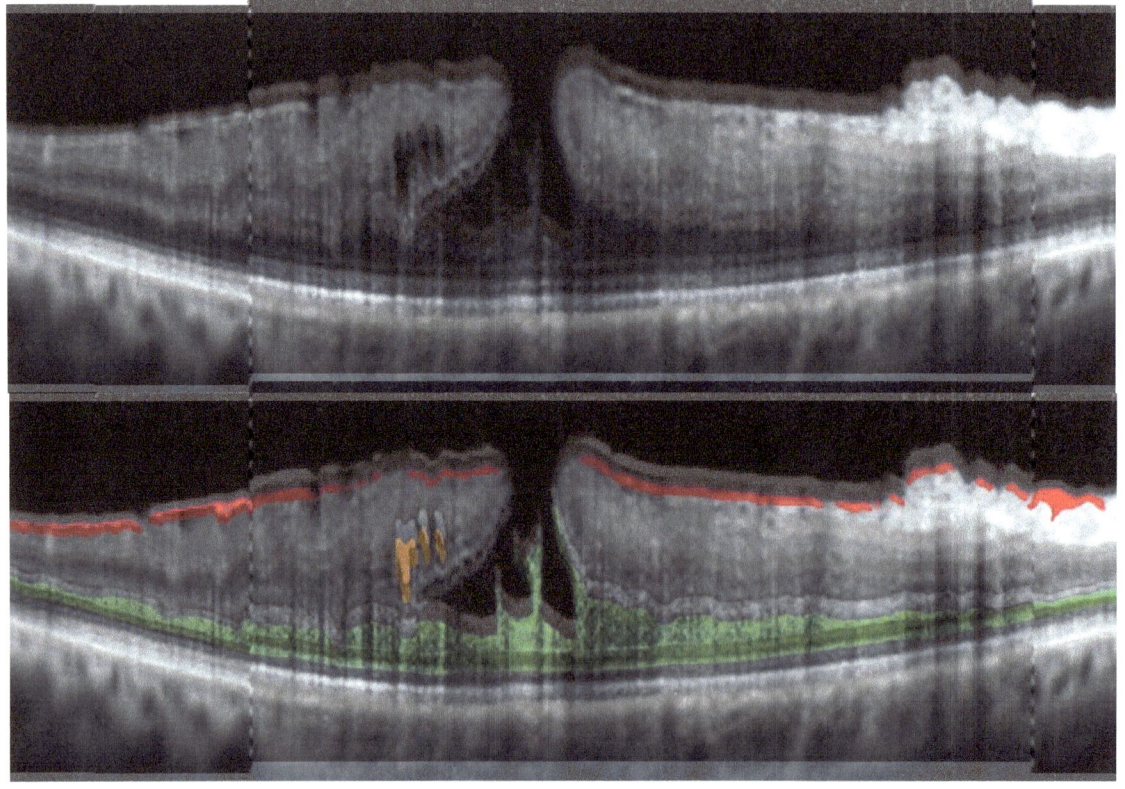

Lamellar Macular Hole

In the OCT image below, the fovea does not have the "typical" appearance of a foveal depression. Looking at the walls of the clivus (the slope of the foveal depression), the ganglion cell layer and inner nuclear layer should gently slope into the foveola and thin out as they approach the foveola, which does not occur in the image below. Normally, at the edge of the foveola the ganglion cell layer is at its closest point (of anywhere in the macula) to the outer plexiform layer. Notice in the image that there is an abrupt discontinuity of the inner nuclear layer (shaded red), and that the ganglion cell layer is still at a distance from the outer plexiform layer. This discontinuity of inner portions of the retina represents a lamellar macular hole:

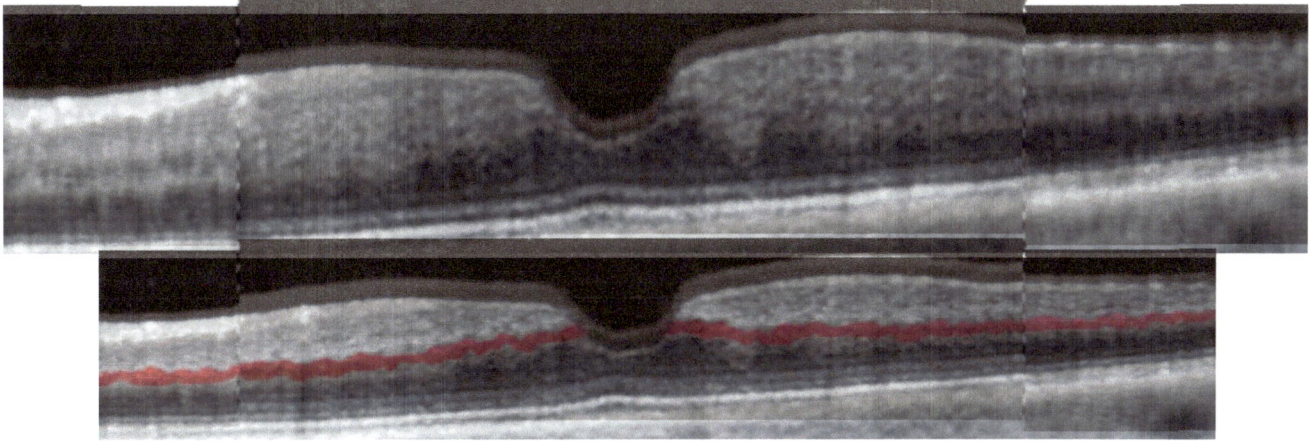

There is frequent association between lamellar macular holes and CME. The images below show a mild CME. Small intraretinal cysts (shaded orange) are forming within the separation (encircled in red) at the inner portion of the outer nuclear layer and the outer portion of the outer plexiform layer. While this case may represent an early state in the process of lamellar hole formation, there is, as yet, no lamellar hole. The ganglion cell layer and inner nuclear layer maintain their slope around the fovea and approach the outer plexiform layer without any discontinuity.

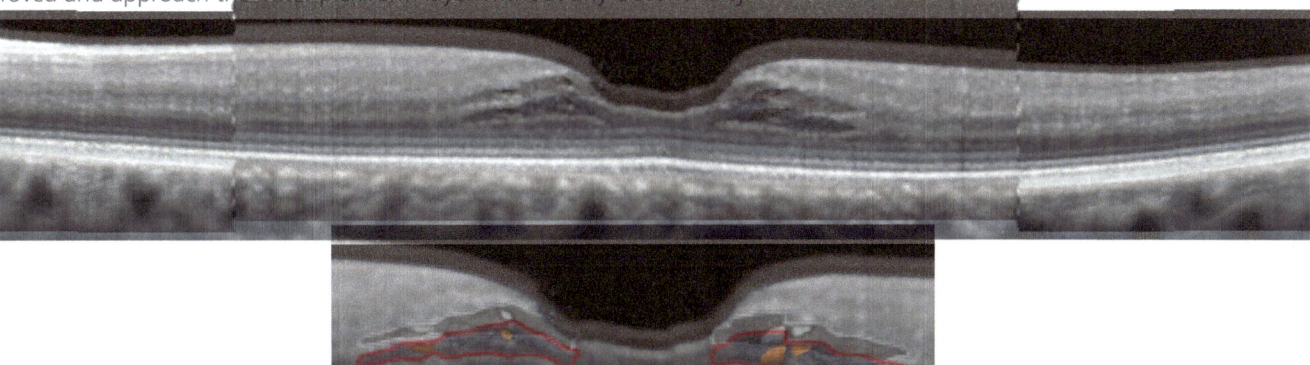

Lamellar macular holes and CME can be subtle. In the case below, the lamellar macular hole (arrow) is associated with an intraretinal cyst (shaded orange).

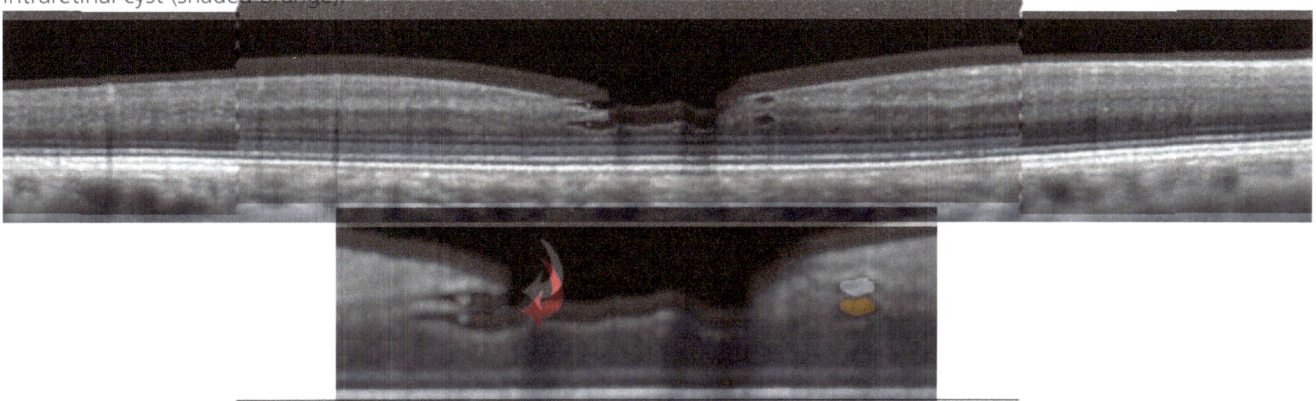

Full-Thickness Macular Hole

The OCT images below show a typical full-thickness macular hole. The hole goes all the way through the retina, exposing the RPE (shaded blue), which appears brighter because the signal reflecting back to the OCT instrument doesn't filter through the retina. The curling of the photoreceptor layers can most easily be identified by tracing the external limiting membrane (shaded yellow) between the photoreceptor nuclear layer and the photoreceptor inner segment myoid zone. Several small intraretinal cysts (shaded orange) can be seen within the inner nuclear layer, between the outer plexiform layer (shaded green) and the inner plexiform layer (shaded red).

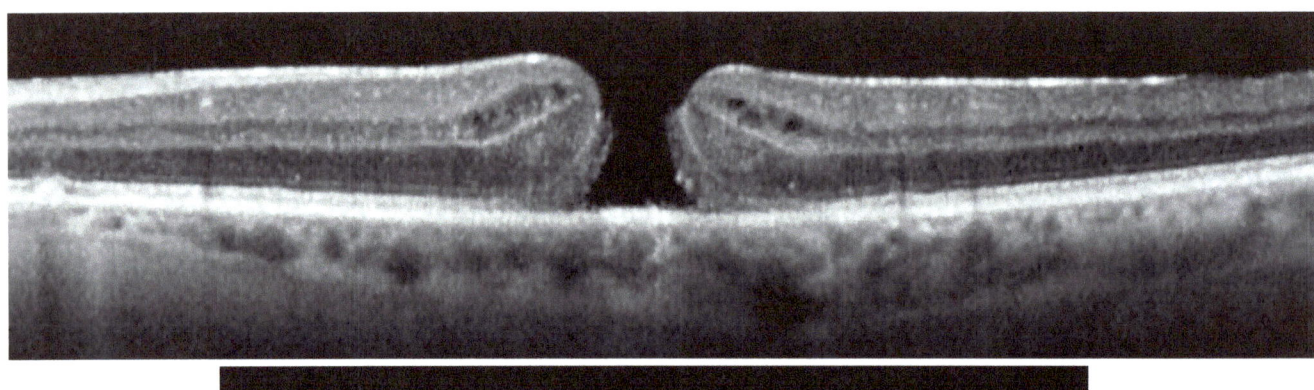

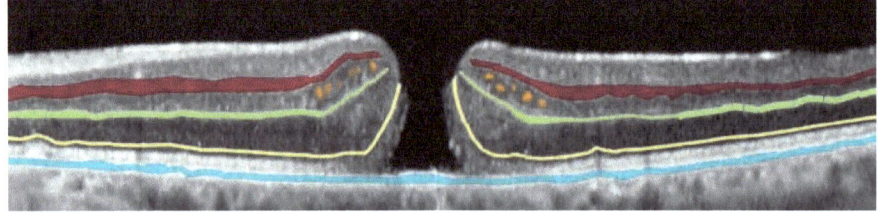

The full-thickness macular hole in the OCT images below has a partial roof (arrow) and the traction from the posterior cortical vitreous (shaded red) is clearly visible. This vitreous traction is believed to be a pathogenic mechanism of the development of macular holes. The hole is full thickness through the retina, as it exposes RPE (shaded yellow). Intraretinal cysts (shaded orange) appear both above and below the outer plexiform layer (shaded green).

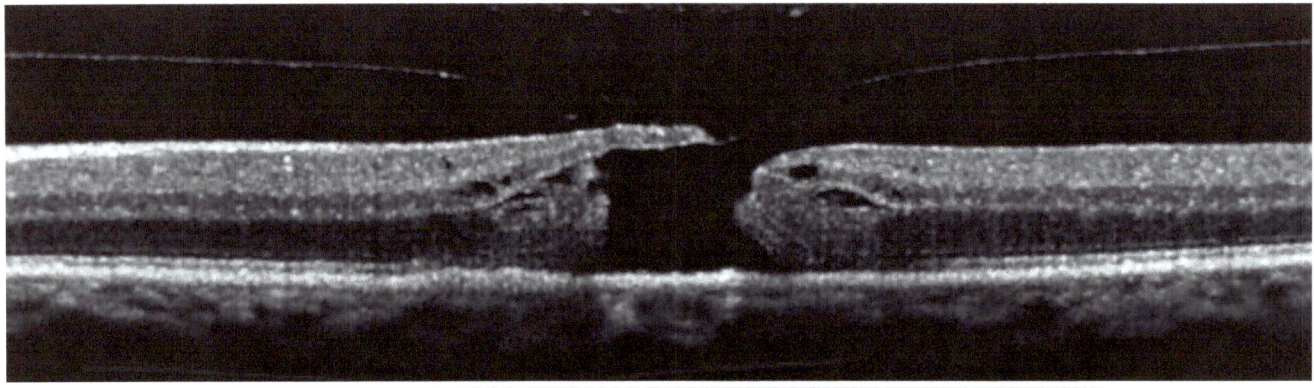

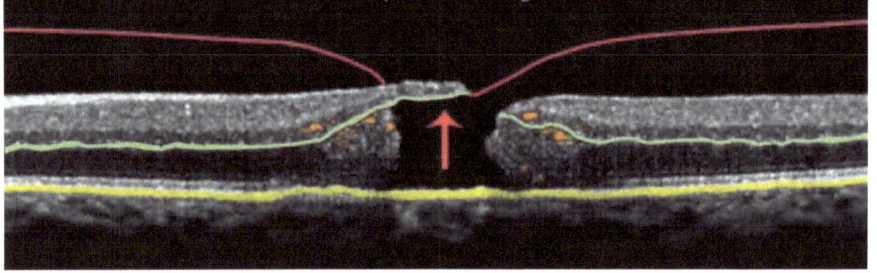

Cystoid Macular Edema

In the OCT images below, large intraretinal cysts (shaded orange) have formed in this patient with CME following cataract extraction. The retina is substantially thickened and small white dots (arrows) likely represent the foci of intraretinal inflammation. These small white dots can often represent the foci of pigment migration, lipid, hemorrhage, or inflammation. Clinical correlation can help in identifying what these white dots represent.

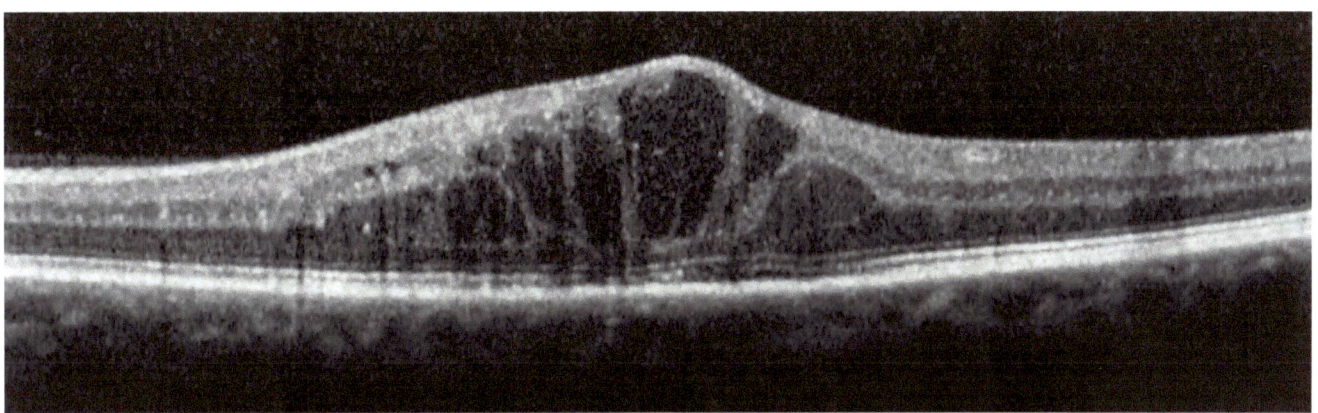

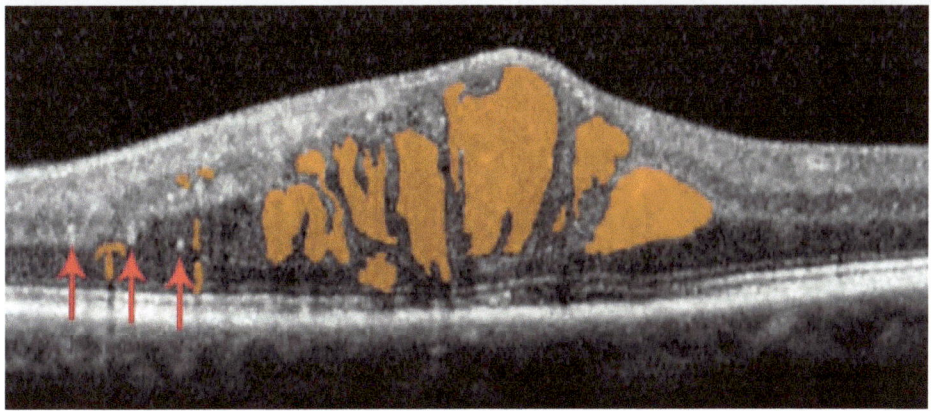

The OCT images below were taken from the same patient after a month of topical therapy. The retinal thickness decreased considerably, and visual acuity improved. Opaque-appearing material (shaded orange), likely cellular debris, is accumulated within one of the intraretinal cysts. Small white dots (arrow), most likely caused by inflammation, are also present.

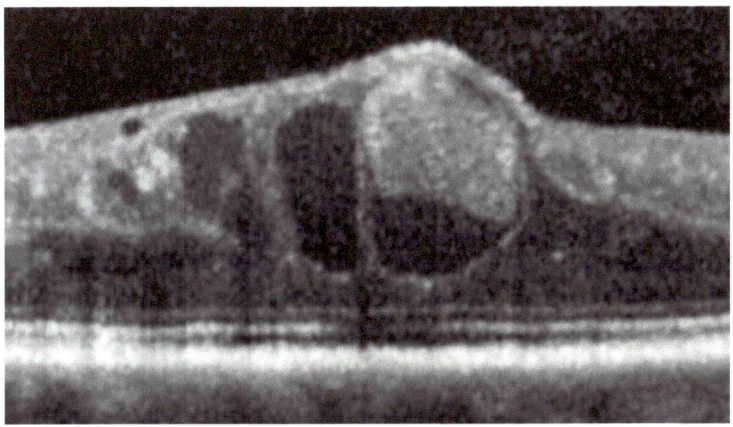
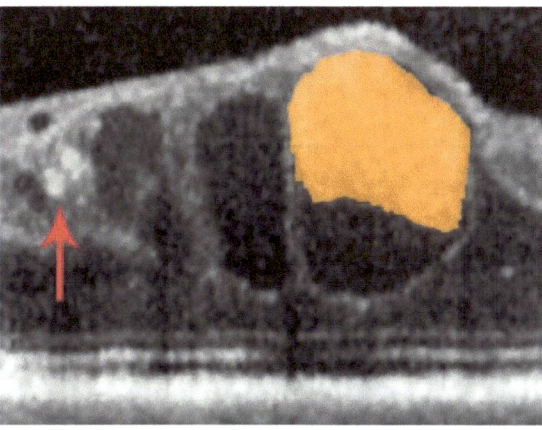

Cystoid Macular Edema

CME: with Subretinal Edema

CME can be associated with subretinal fluid. In the OCT images below, the patient has macular edema with intraretinal cysts (shaded orange), as well as subretinal fluid (shaded blue). The subretinal fluid is located between the RPE (shaded green) and the photoreceptor band, which can be identified by tracing the ellipsoid zone of the photoreceptors (shaded red). This patient presents with wet macular degeneration with choroidal neovascularization causing both the cystoid macular edema and the subretinal fluid.

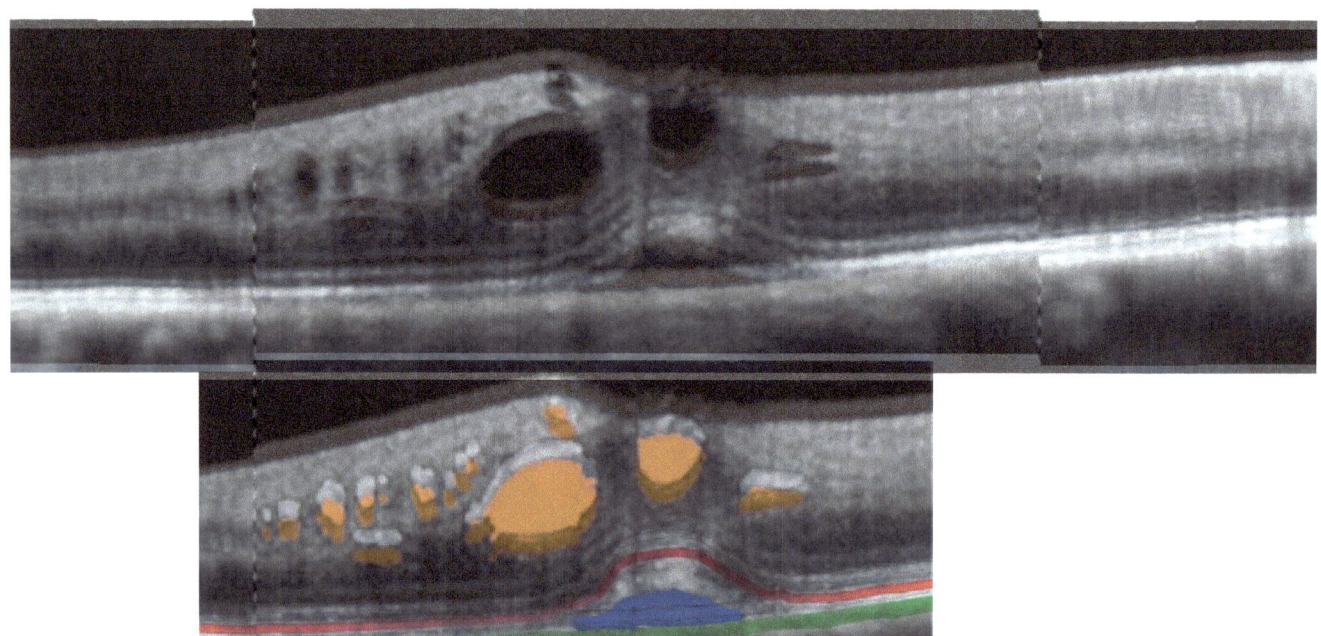

In the OCT images below, the intraretinal cysts (shaded orange) are mostly concentrated in the inner nuclear layer but are also apparent in the outer nuclear layer and the ganglion cell layer. There is also a small pocket of subretinal fluid beneath the macula, separating the photoreceptors from the RPE.

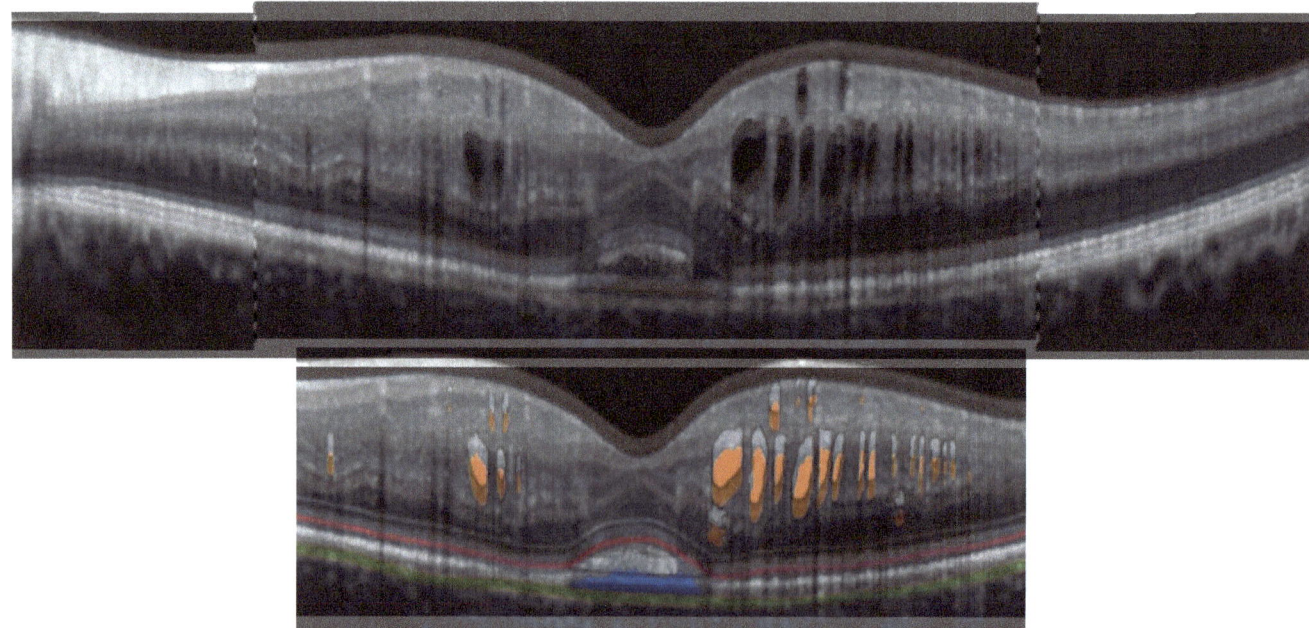

Cysts, Exudates, and Outer Retinal Holes

Small intraretinal cysts (arrows) are present near the fovea in the two patient images below. However, there is no leakage on fluorescein angiography. These intraretinal cysts represent cystic formation from previous resolved macular edema without any current active leakage. Not all cysts on OCT mean active leakage.

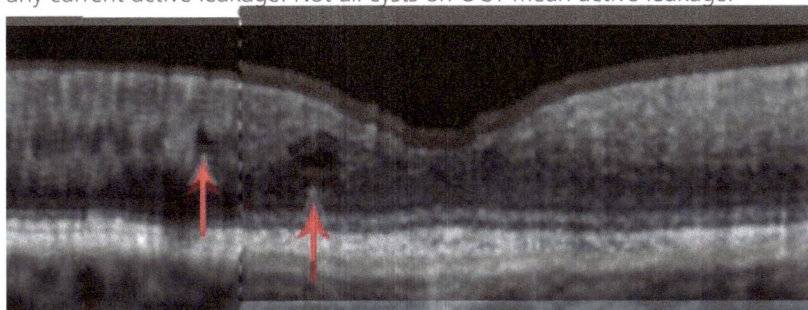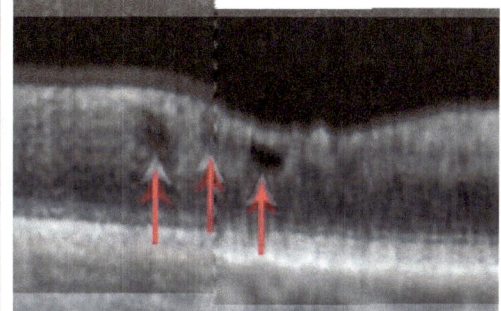

In the patient below, the OCT images appear to show intraretinal cysts. However, in the left image, notice that the "cyst" (arrow) is in the photoreceptor layer of the outer retina and that there is no associated thickening of the retina. This pattern is not a cyst but an outer retinal hole, which has resulted from long standing solar retinopathy. Photoreceptors are lost due to damage from sun gazing, resulting in the empty space: the outer retinal hole. To the right of (nasal to) the outer retinal hole, the bright line representing the ellipsoid zone of the photoreceptors abruptly ends, and to the left of (temporal to) the outer retinal hole, there is disorganization of the outer retinal layers. In the image to the right, the chronic solar retinopathy has resulted in an outer retinal hole (arrow) as well as an inner retinal hole that represents loss of inner retinal neurons and supporting cells. The inner retinal hole is roofed by an intact external limiting membrane and posterior hyaloid (arrowhead).

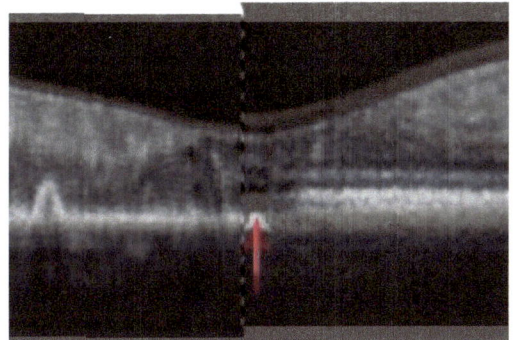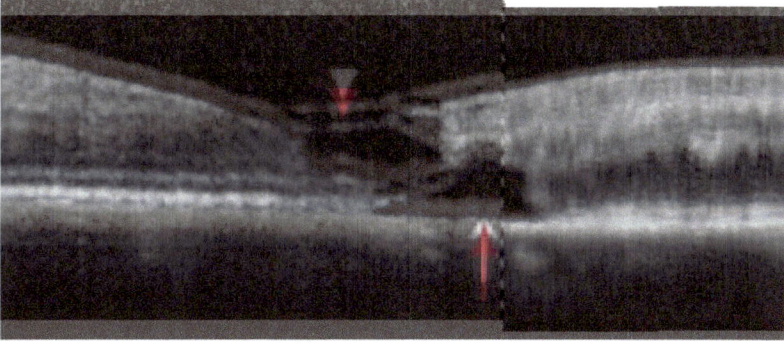

In the OCT image of the patient below, white intraretinal dots and larger aggregates (arrows), represent lipid or hard exudates. This patient has non-proliferative diabetic retinopathy with clinically-significant macular edema. Hard exudates are visible adjacent to the fovea on fundoscopy. Notice the shadowing effect from these hard exudates on the OCT. The image shows intraretinal cysts within the outer nuclear layer (outlined in orange) as well as a somewhat thickened retina (doubled headed arrow). Within the retina, white dots and aggregates can often represent foci of pigment migration, lipid or hard exudate, hemorrhage, or inflammation. Clinical correlation can help in identifying what these white dots and aggregates represent.

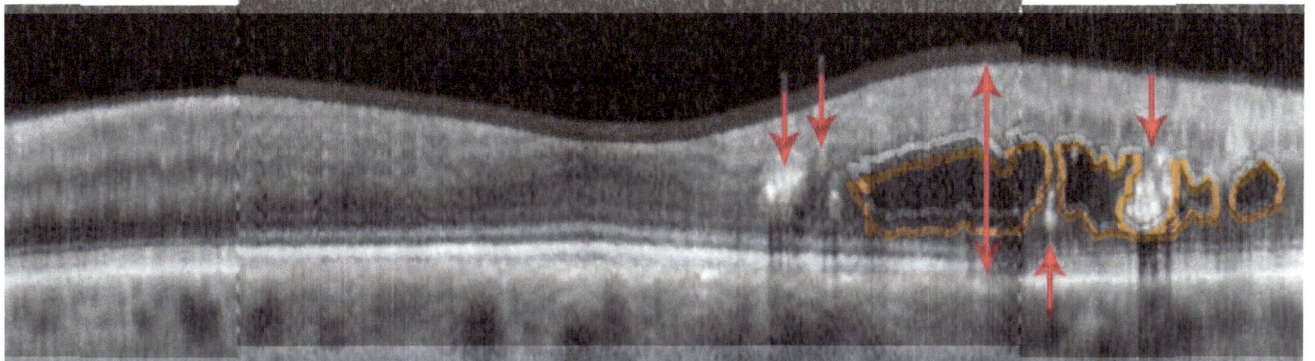

Diabetic Macular Edema

In the OCT image below of a patient with non-proliferative diabetic retinopathy, there is a very small area of retinal thickening (double-headed arrow) immediately adjacent to the center of the fovea, and there is an intraretinal cyst (outlined in orange) visible on OCT as well as on clinical examination via contact-lens biomicroscopy. On fluorescein angiography, there are two leaking microaneurysms within this area and the patient's acuity was 20/25. Although the edema is very mild, this patient has clinically-significant macular edema. When the patient received three spots of light laser photocoagulation, the edema resolved and visual acuity improved to 20/20.

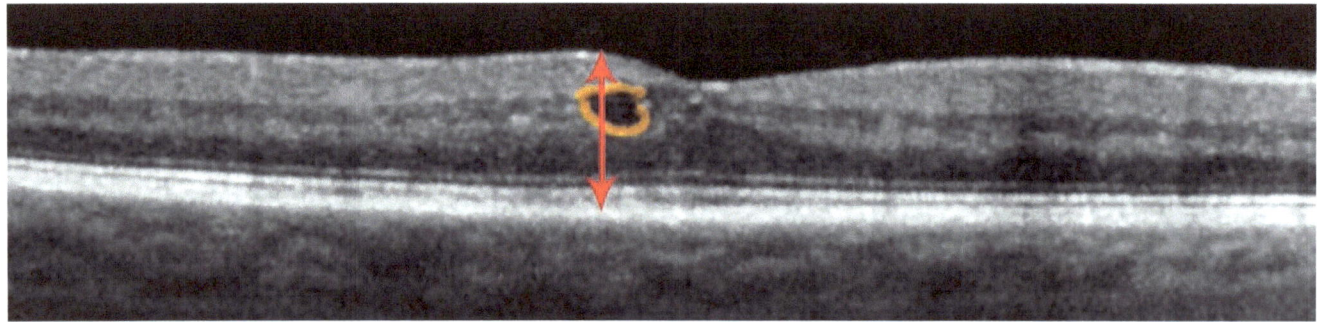

In the image below, the patient presents with proliferative diabetic retinopathy with clinically-significant macular edema. There is a moderate amount of intraretinal cysts (outlined in orange) and the retina is thickened in this area.

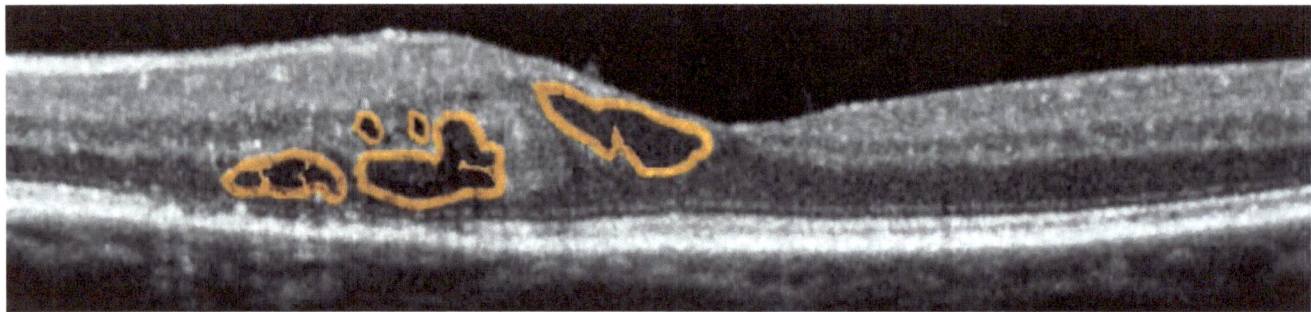

Below, the edema in this patient with non-proliferative diabetic retinopathy resembles non-diabetic CME. The numerous cysts in this patient with diabetic cystoid macular edema are located in multiple layers within the retina. The increased brightness of the outer retina within the fovea (arrow) is due to the increased transmission of light from the OCT system through the large translucent foveal cyst; this phenomenon is the opposite of shadowing.

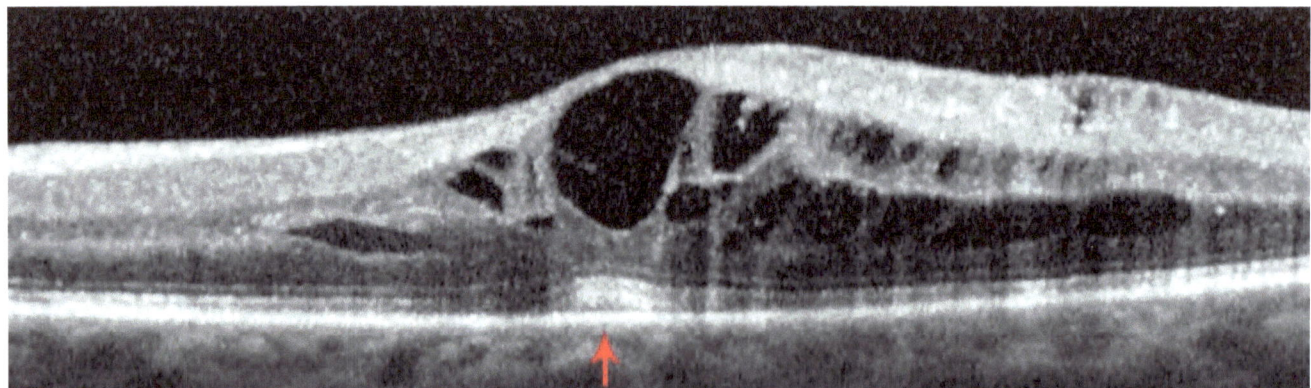

Dry Macular Degeneration

In dry age-related macular degeneration (AMD), drusen can be identified as irregularities generally appearing within the level of the RPE (shaded green) on OCT (though the irregularities may be above, below, or within the RPE). In each case below, the ellipsoid zone of the photoreceptors (shaded red) remains above the drusen, though it clearly undulates up and down as it layers on top of the wavy RPE and drusen. In some areas, the ellipsoid zone is obscured, suggesting possible loss of photoreceptors in these spaces (areas of discontinuity in shaded red line). The loss may be complete, or more likely partial with photoreceptor degeneration.

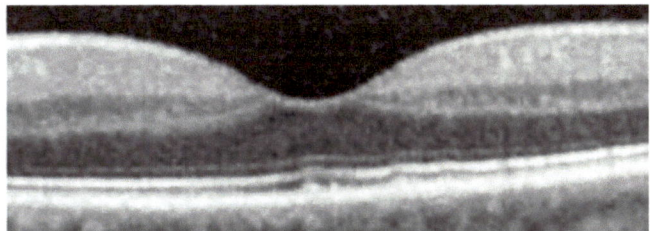 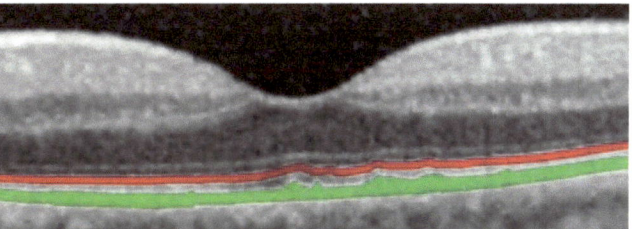

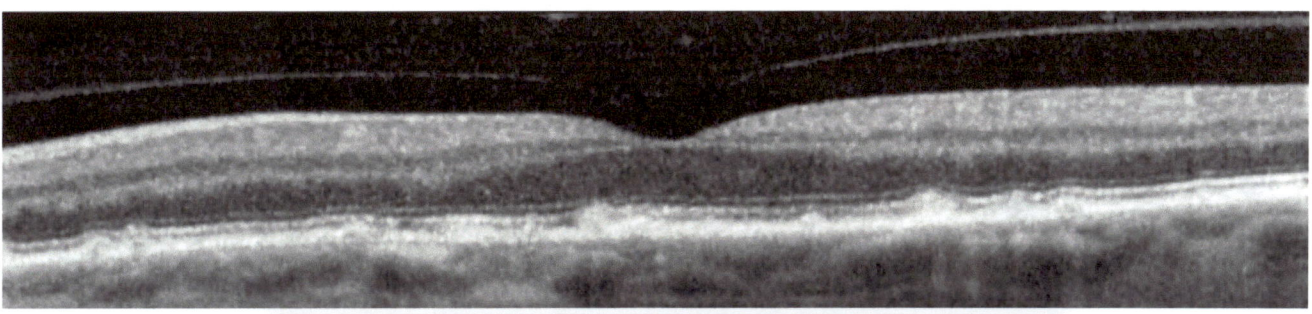

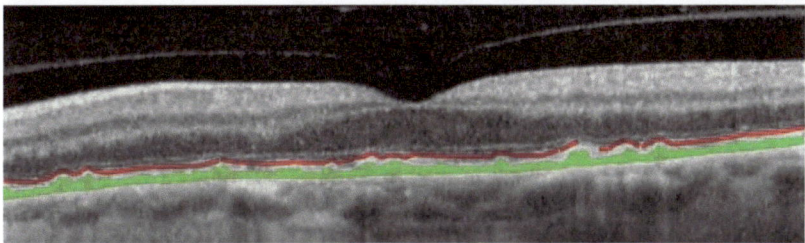

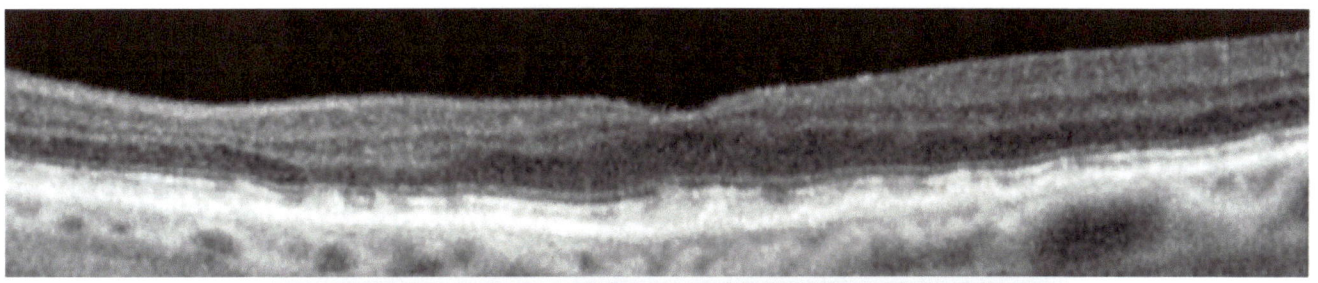

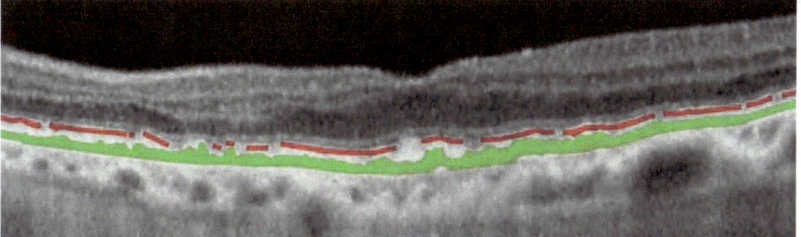

Dry Macular Degeneration

AMD: with Drusenoid Pigment Epithelial Detachments

When the "debris" (shaded orange) in dry AMD is clearly seen below elevated portions of the RPE (shaded green), then RPE is considered to be "detached", or elevated above the underlying choriocapillaris and choroid. Bruch's membrane (shaded light blue), a portion of which is the basement membrane of the RPE, is often easily identifiable in these elevated areas. The "debris" is referred to as drusenoid, as it often resembles drusen clinically, and these areas are called drusenoid RPE detachments or drusenoid pigment epithelial detachments (drusenoid PEDs).¹ In some areas, the photoreceptor ellipsoid zone (shaded red) is obscured, suggesting possible partial or complete loss of photoreceptors (areas of discontinuity shaded in red). Below are two separate cases of dry AMD with drusenoid PEDs.

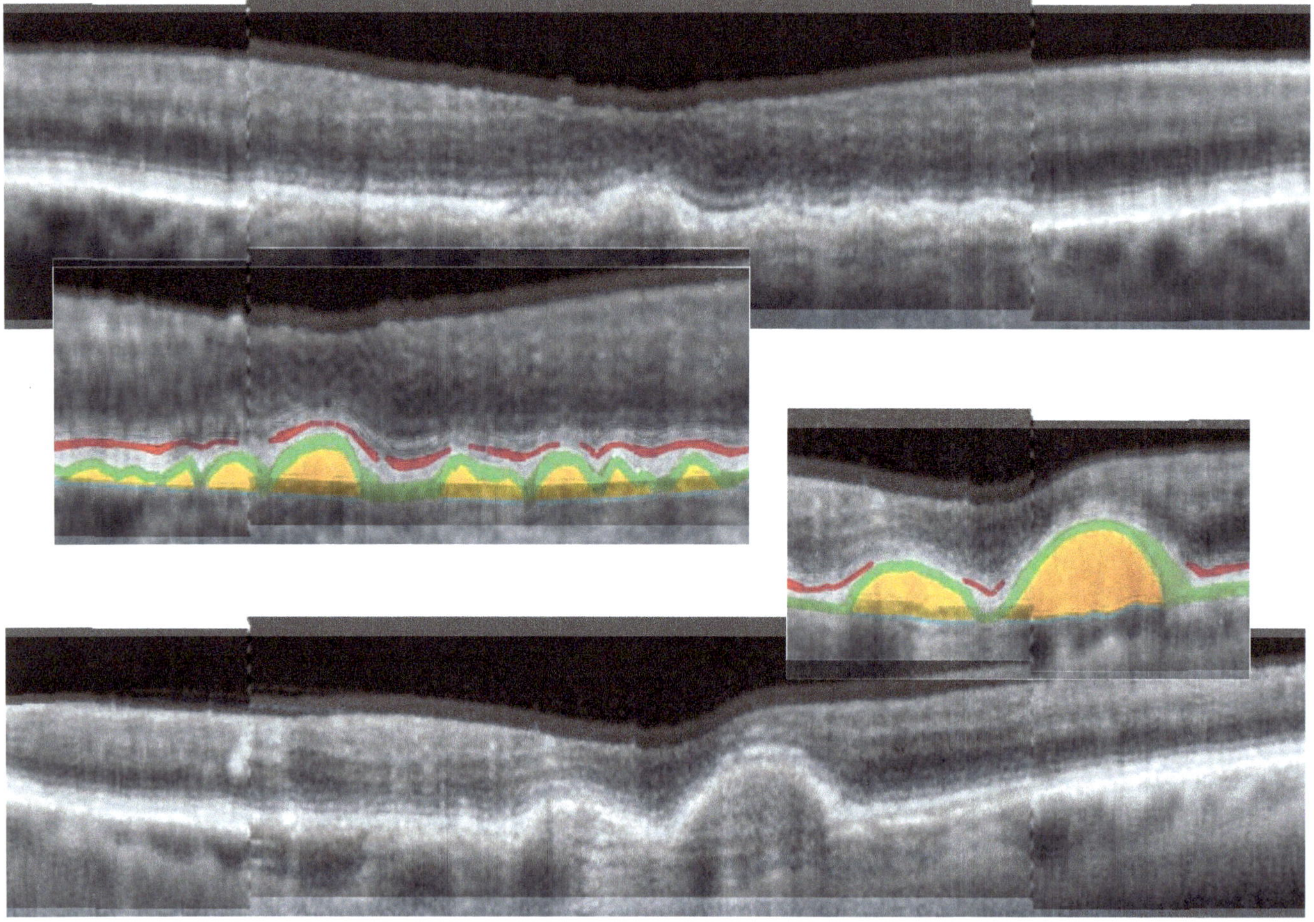

In the patient below, the central nodularity may suggest a drusenoid PED, but the RPE (shaded green) is in a normal position overlying the choriocapillaris and choroid. Since the "debris" is above the RPE, this is classified as a large central druse (shaded orange).¹ The photoreceptor layer is evidenced by the ellipsoid zone (shaded red) and is overlying the druse.

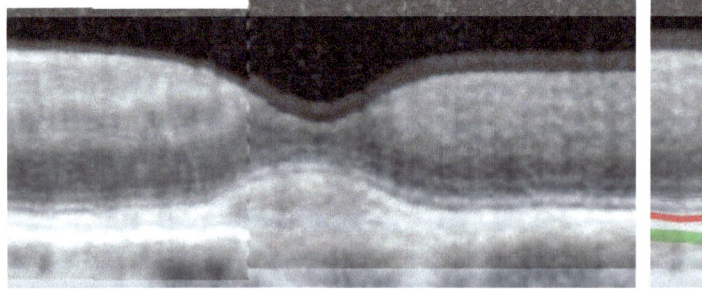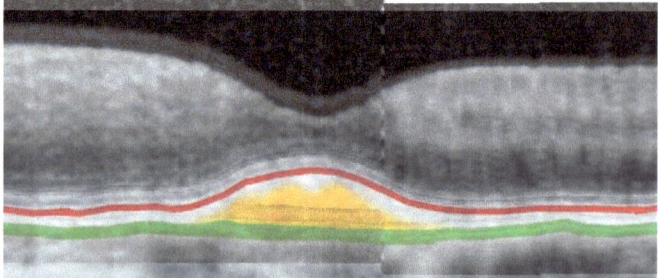

¹ See table describing drusen on page 23

Characteristics of Drusen

Comparisons of OCT, Clinical Examination, and Histopathology

OCT Terminology	OCT Appearance	Clinical Terminology	Clinical Appearance	Comments	Histological Appearance
Drusen above the RPE.	Reflective material located between the RPE and the retina, with minimal distortion of overlying retina.	Subretinal drusenoid deposits.	Varying clinical descriptions are found in the clinical literature, but these drusen are commonly described as appearing to be small, soft drusen with poorly defined or indiscrete margins. Unlike typical soft drusen, these drusen are less visible under typical slit-lamp biomicroscopy with a standard light source, and are best viewed in the one or more of the under red-free light or blue light. Also, unlike typical soft drusen, these drusen tend to be but do not always display an articular pattern or network.	Subretinal drusenoid deposits. The clinical term "subretinal drusenoid deposits" is a newer term for reticular pseudodrusen.	Histopathologically, these drusen too soft drusen, except that they are located above rather than below the RPE.
		Reticular pseudodrusen.		Reticular pseudodrusen are sometimes referred to as subretinal drusenoid deposits.	
Drusen at the level of the RPE.	RPE lifts tending, irregular, or often lumpy.	Hard drusen.	Drusen with sharp margins; small (< 64 microns) to medium (64-125 microns) in size.	On OCT, these hard drusen appear to be located within the RPE; however, on many occasions, these drusen are actually located beneath the RPE in both cases, the material is within the RPE.	Histopathologically, hard drusen are commonly identified as accumulations of material underneath the RPE (ie, these hard drusen areas of RPE accumulation of material along the inner aspect of Bruch's membrane (basal linear deposits) and/or between the RPE and the RPE's basement membrane (basal laminar deposits). This type of hard drusen is histopathologically referred to as a nodular drusen. In both cases, the material is accumulated within the RPE and referred to as a lipoidal or lipoidal degeneration of RPE.
		Soft drusen.	Drusen with indistinct margins; medium (64-125 microns) in size.	Soft drusen are actually the accumulation of material underneath the RPE with the resulting pigment epithelial detachments.	Histopathologically, soft drusen are localized areas of pigment epithelial detachments with accumulation of basal laminar deposits (material located underneath the RPE) and/or basal linear deposits (material located within the RPE's basement membrane).
Drusenoid detachment or RPE's basement membrane (drusenoid PEDs).	Reflective material located beneath the RPE and above the RPE's basement membrane.	Soft confluent drusen.	Drusen with indistinct margins; that are often larger (>125 microns) in size and appear amorphous in shape and extent.	Often, soft drusen may fall in between these clinical categories of soft drusen and confluent drusen; it is often difficult to make a distinction between the two clinical subtypes.	Often, soft drusen (material located between the RPE and the RPE's basement membrane).
		Cuticular drusen.	Small to medium nodular appearing drusen, that have a generally rounded shape and appear to be elevated because of their localized RPE detachment.	Cuticular drusen are sometimes called basal laminar drusen.	Consists of basal laminar deposits in and/or basal linear deposits (see above), with localized pigment epithelial detachments. These drusen have a smaller in size and appear nodular.
		Basal laminar drusen.		A histopathologic term for basal laminar drusen. The term basal laminar drusen should not to be confused with basal laminar deposits (material located between the RPE and the RPE's basement membrane).	
		Drusenoid pigment epithelial detachments.	Large, soft, and confluent drusen, with or without RPE is visibly detached.	Clinically, these larger soft drusen are called drusenoid pigment epithelial detachments, though histopathologically, they are defined to be all the same.	Consists of basal laminar deposits and/or basal linear deposits (see above) with localized pigment epithelial detachment.

Dry Macular Degeneration

AMD and Geographic Atrophy

This patient with AMD and resolved choroidal neovascularization retained 20/30 visual acuity after multiple intravitreal injections of an anti-VEGF agent. The images below do not reveal any subretinal fluid, subretinal hemorrhage, intraretinal cysts, retinal thickening, or subretinal fibrosis. There is some mild residual pigment epithelial detachment, visible between the RPE (shaded red) and Bruch's membrane, a portion of which is the RPE cells' basement membrane (shaded green).

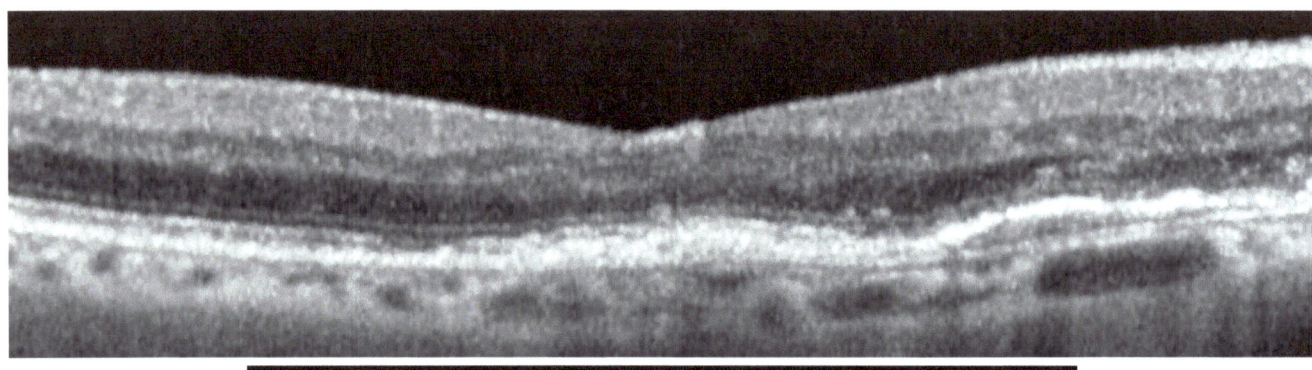

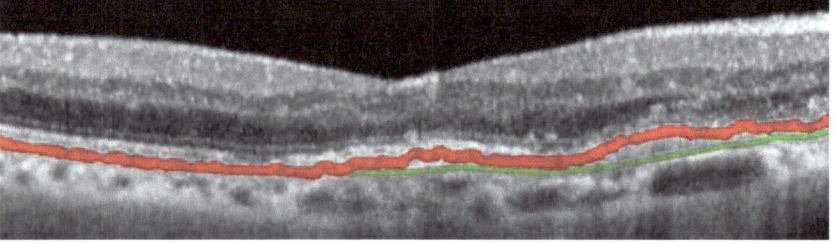

The patient below with dry macular degeneration also presents with geographic atrophy (GA). Upon clinical examination, it appears that the retina is thinned and the RPE is lost within this area of GA (double-headed arrow). The RPE (shaded purple), along with the ellipsoid zone of the photoreceptors (shaded blue), the external limiting membrane (shaded yellow) and the outer nuclear layer, which is the photoreceptor nuclei (shaded green) all abruptly end over the area of geographic atrophy, suggesting loss of the RPE as well as loss of photoreceptors. The inner nuclear layer (shaded red) remains a continuous layer stretching across the area of GA. In these OCT images, the retina also appears thinner. The increased brightness of the choroid at the area of GA (double-headed arrow) is due to the increased transmission and reflectance of light from the OCT system through the GA; this phenomenon is the opposite of shadowing.

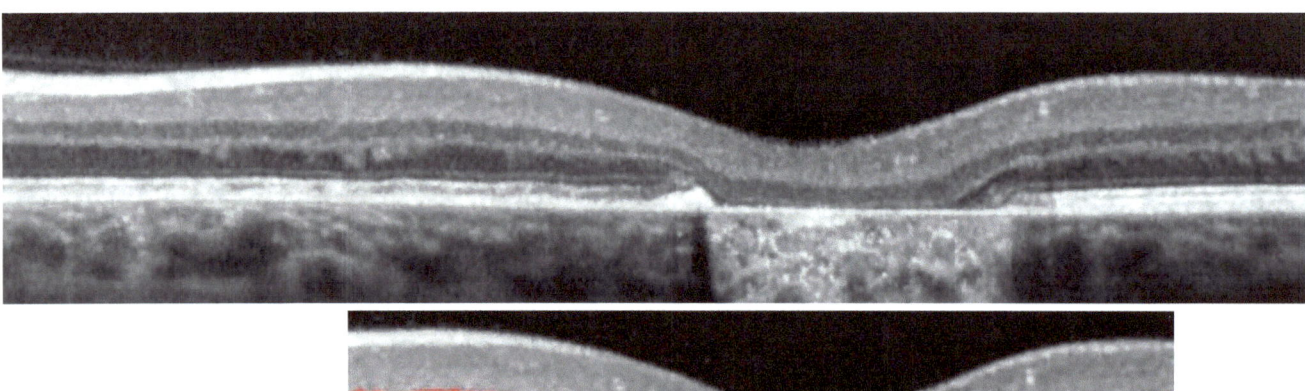

Wet Macular Degeneration

In wet AMD, the choroidal neovascularization may be underneath the RPE (shaded light blue). In the case below, the RPE is detached or elevated above the underlying choriocapillaris and choroid. No "material" is visible within this PED (shaded orange). Bruch's membrane, a portion of which is the RPE's basement membrane (shaded pink) is visible. On fluorescein and high-speed indocyanine green (ICG) angiography, there is leakage suggestive of "occult" or sub-RPE choroidal neovascularization. Overlying the PED, the photoreceptor ellipsoid zone (shaded yellow) is obscured, suggesting possible partial atrophy or degeneration of photoreceptors in these areas (note the discontinuity in the shaded yellow line). The presence of the outer nuclear layer (shaded red), though varying in thickness, and the presence of the external limiting membrane (green line) indicate that some photoreceptor components remain present.

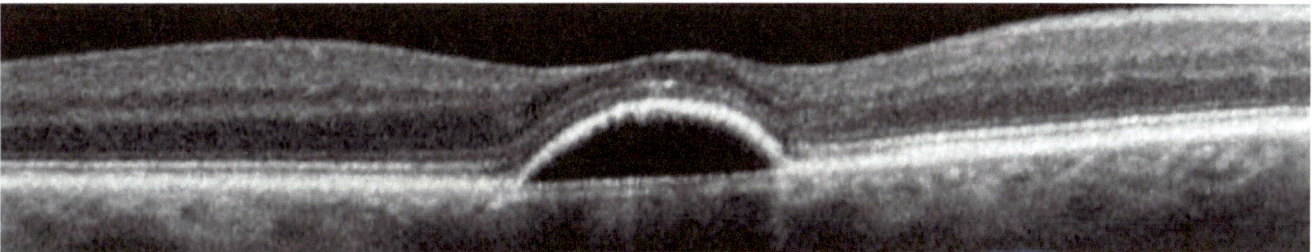

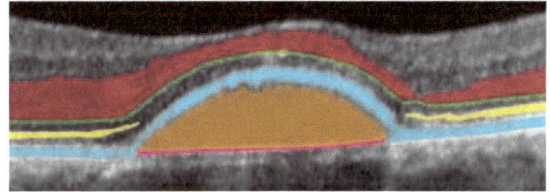

In the case below, choroidal neovascularization is present beneath the RPE (shaded red), with some material seen within the PED (shaded orange). Bruch's membrane (shaded green), is easily identifiable. On fluorescein and high-speed ICG angiography, shows leakage consistent with "occult" or sub-RPE choroidal neovascularization. Again, overlying the PED, the photoreceptor ellipsoid zone (shaded yellow) is obscured, suggesting possible partial atrophy or degeneration of photoreceptors in these areas (discontinuity in shaded yellow line). Small white dots (arrows) likely represent the foci of intraretinal inflammation in this patient; a larger one (arrowhead) is likely migrated pigment. The identity of these white dots is often not readily apparent on OCT and must be determined based on clinical examination in conjunction with the assessment of OCT scans.

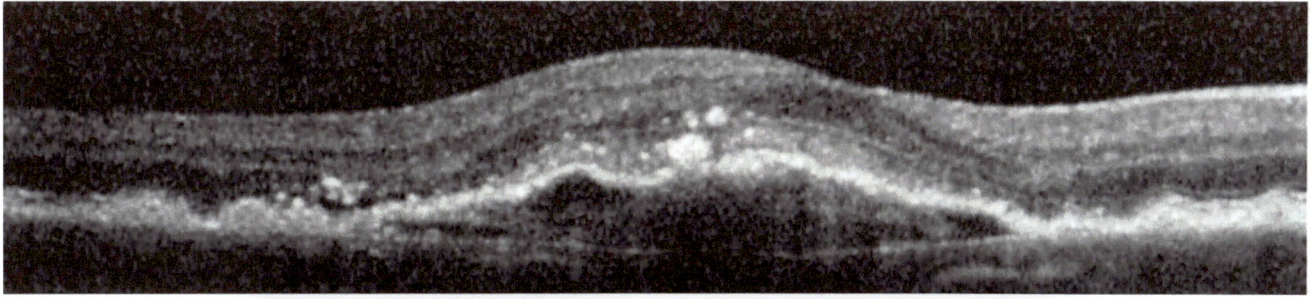

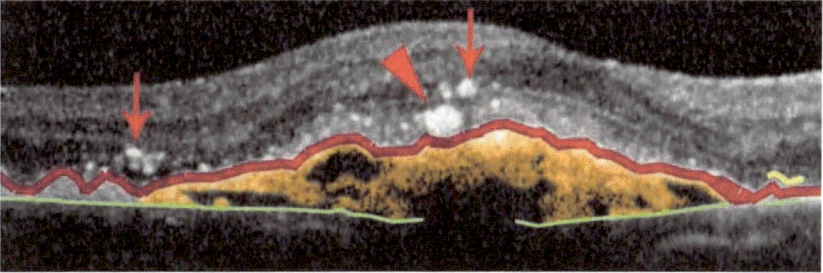

Wet Macular Degeneration

CNV: Subretinal Fluid, Pigment Epithelial Detachment

The subretinal fluid (shaded orange) and the PED (shaded purple) can be identified in the images below by tracing the RPE (shaded green) in this patient presenting with wet AMD. The photoreceptors can be located by tracing the photoreceptor ellipsoid zone of the photoreceptors (shaded red). By fluorescein angiography, the choroidal neovascularization appears predominately "classic". The images below are adjacent OCT cross-sections parallel to each other, through the fovea (above) and adjacent to the fovea (below).

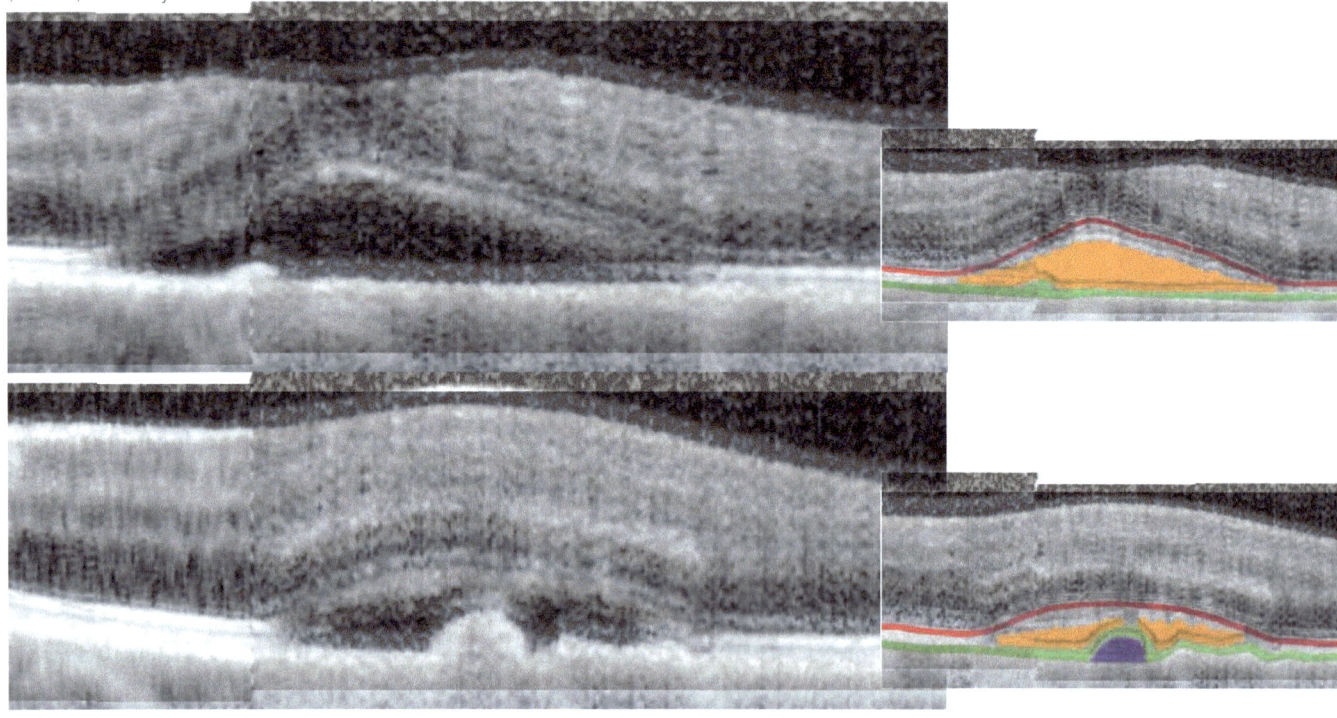

In the upper OCT image of the patient below, a small PED (shaded purple) is visible underneath the RPE (shaded green) along with a mild amount of subretinal fluid (shaded orange). The bottom image is an OCT cross-section adjacent and parallel to the top image. In the bottom image, the PED is not visible, but the subretinal fluid should raise concerns. The patient has choroidal neovascularization, identified by fluorescein and high-speed ICG angiography.

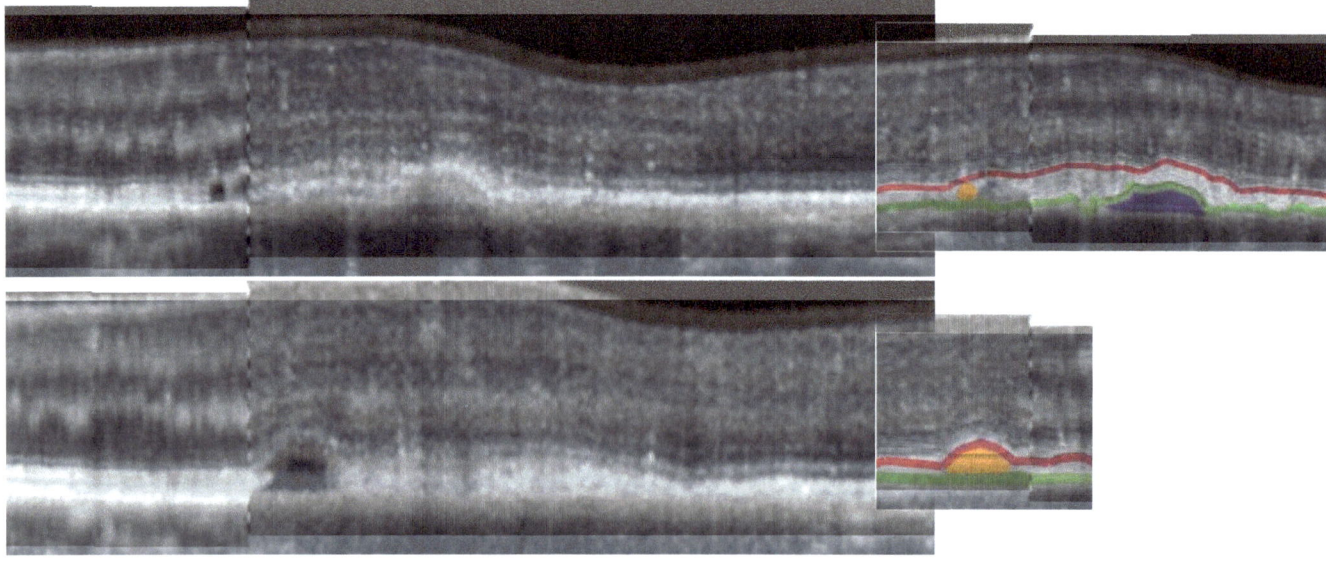

Wet Macular Degeneration

CNV: Cysts, Subretinal Fluid

In the cases below of AMD with choroidal neovascularization, the RPE (shaded red) and Bruch's membrane (shaded green) can be used to trace the large PEDs. Figure 1 shows subretinal fluid (shaded orange); Figure 2 includes macular cysts (shaded in blue); and Figure 3 contains both subretinal fluid and macular cysts.

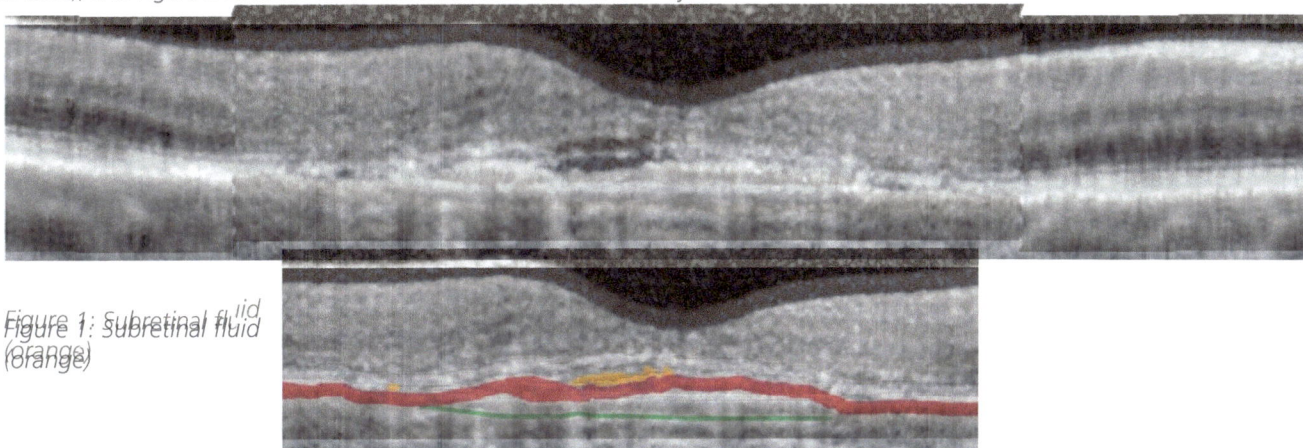

Figure 1: Subretinal fluid (orange)

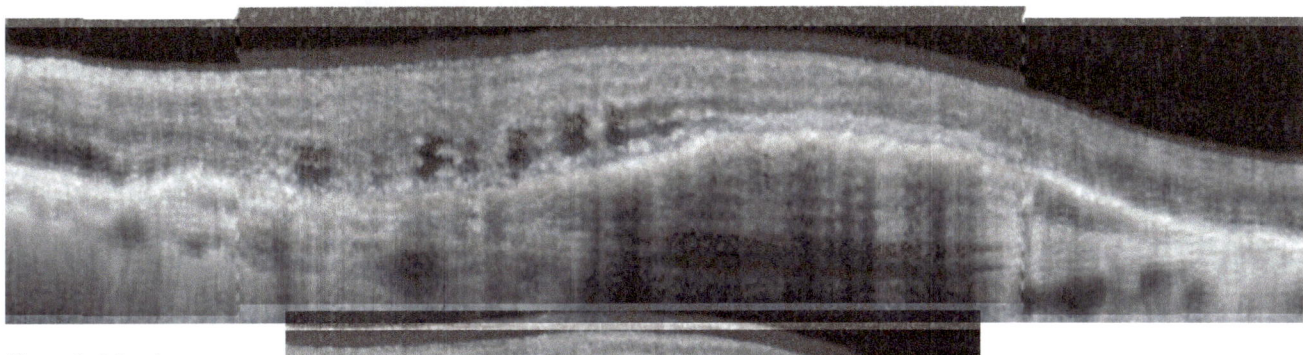

Figure 2: Macular cysts (blue)

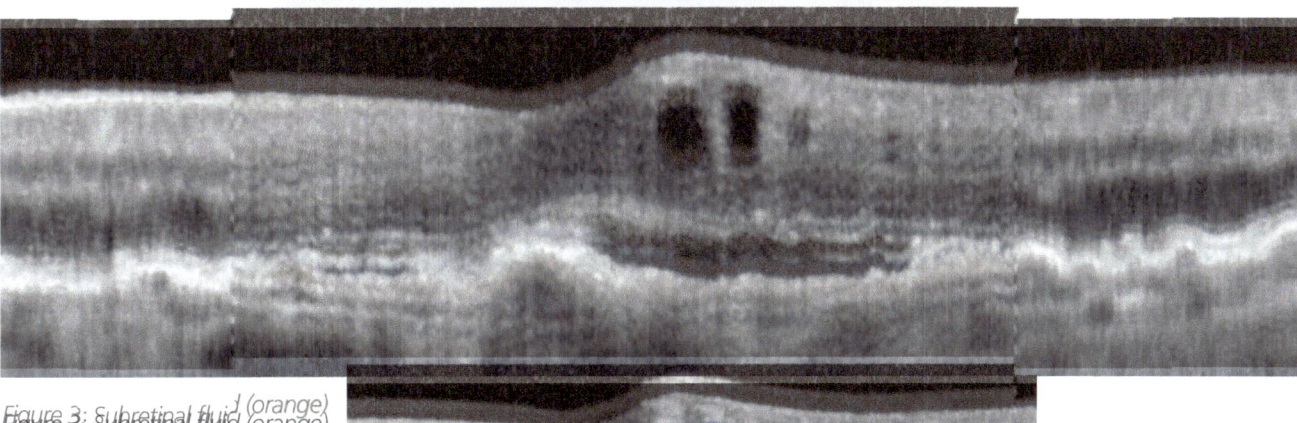

Figure 3: Subretinal fluid (orange) and macular cysts (blue)

Wet Macular Degeneration

CNV: Subretinal Hemorrhage

In the images below, the patient presents with AMD, choroidal neovascularization, a PED, and a subretinal hemorrhage (shaded orange) located above the RPE (shaded red) and below the retina.

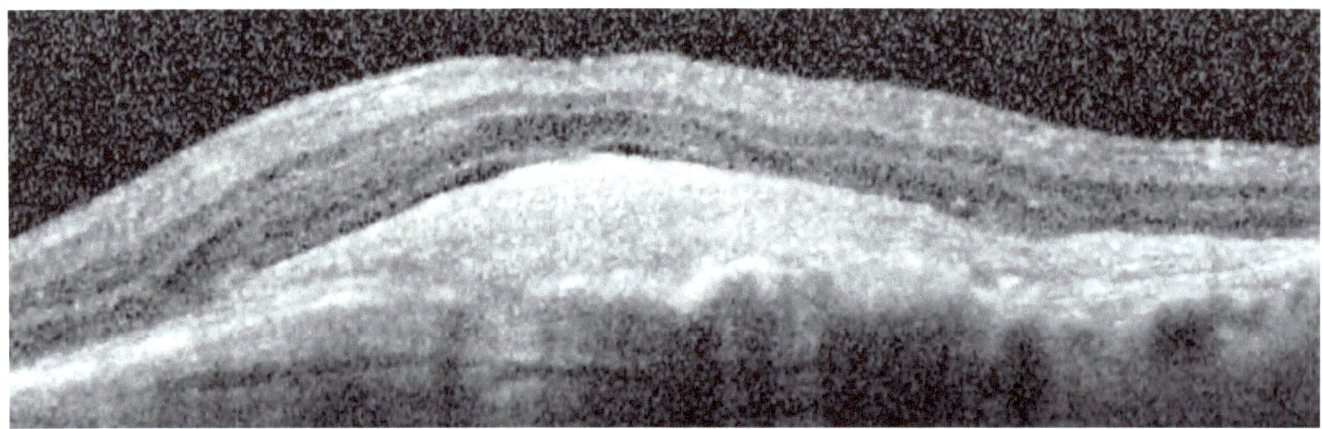

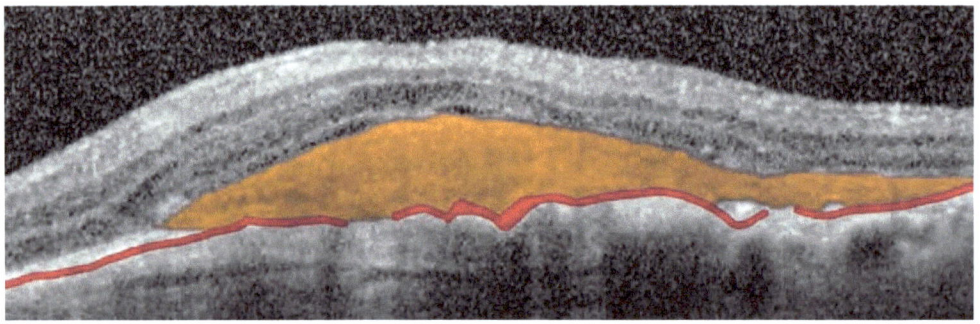

In the OCT image of the patient below, the subretinal hemorrhage (shaded orange) and the subretinal fluid (shaded blue) are located above the RPE (shaded yellow) and below the retina. The loss of the ellipsoid zone of the photoreceptors (shaded green) and the external limiting membrane (shaded red), signifies degeneration and atrophy of the photoreceptors.

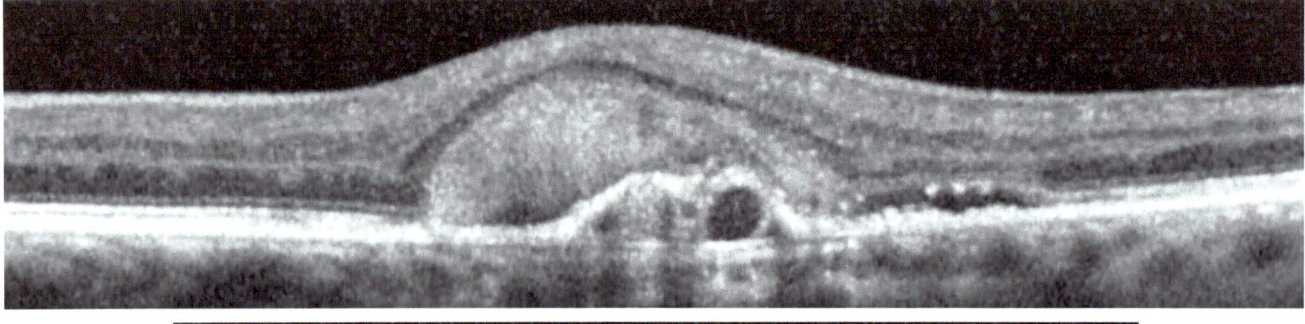

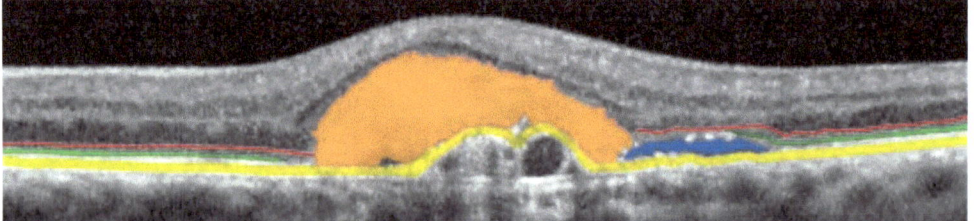

Wet Macular Degeneration

CNV: Disciform Scarring

In end-stage AMD with choroidal neovascularization as seen in the images below, early subretinal fibrosis progresses to disciform scarring. The subretinal fibrosis (shaded orange) has a dense white appearance due to the high reflectivity of the material. There is likely degeneration and atrophy of the photoreceptors, both above and adjacent to the subretinal fibrosis, as evidenced by loss of the ellipsoid zone of the photoreceptors (shaded green). Tracing the outer plexiform layer (shaded red) can assist in identifying the structures remaining within the retina.

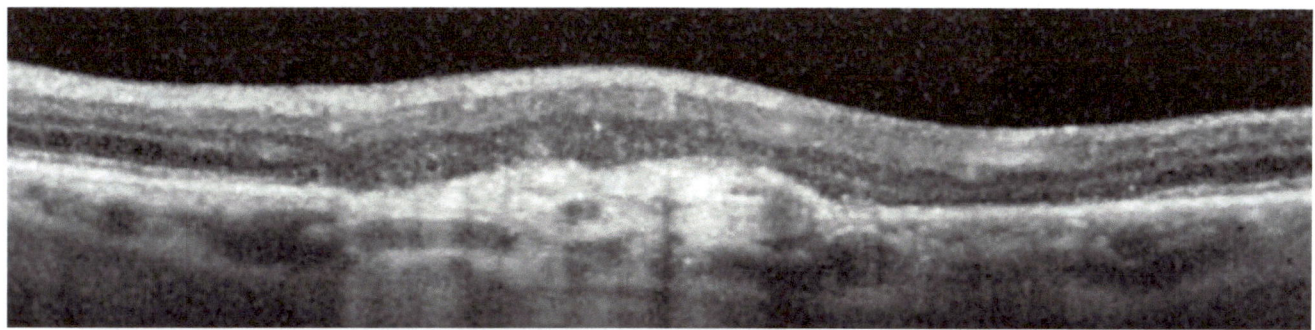

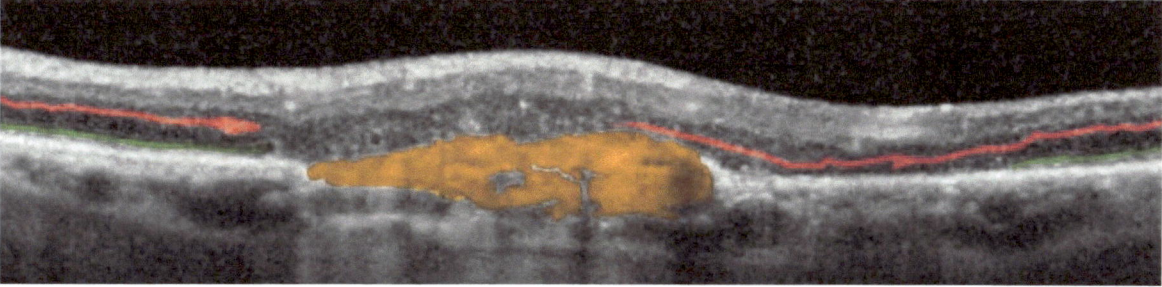

In the case below, the subretinal fibrosis (shaded orange) is quite dense, and the retina demonstrates a pattern called "intraretinal tubulation". Notice the scrolling appearance of the outer plexiform layer (shaded red) and tube-like structures (shaded green) mostly within the photoreceptor bands. Many of the bands comprising the photoreceptors are absent or disorganized.

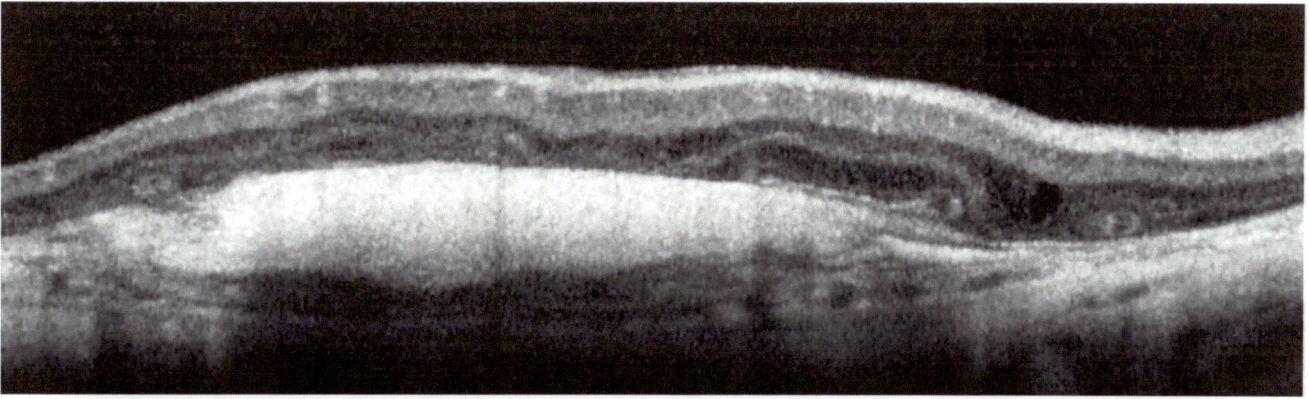

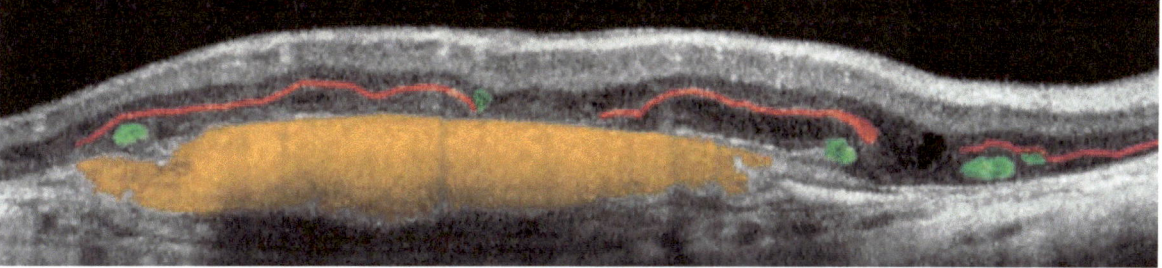

Central Serous Chorioretinopathy

Central serous chorioretinopathy may mimic AMD. In the images below, subretinal fluid (shaded green) is observed in active disease. Small white spots (red arrows) within the retina likely represent foci of inflammation. This OCT image was taken through the inferotemporal arcade near the optic nerve head. Notice that the RNFL (shaded purple) is thick and contains two vessels (arrowheads) with shadowing effects.

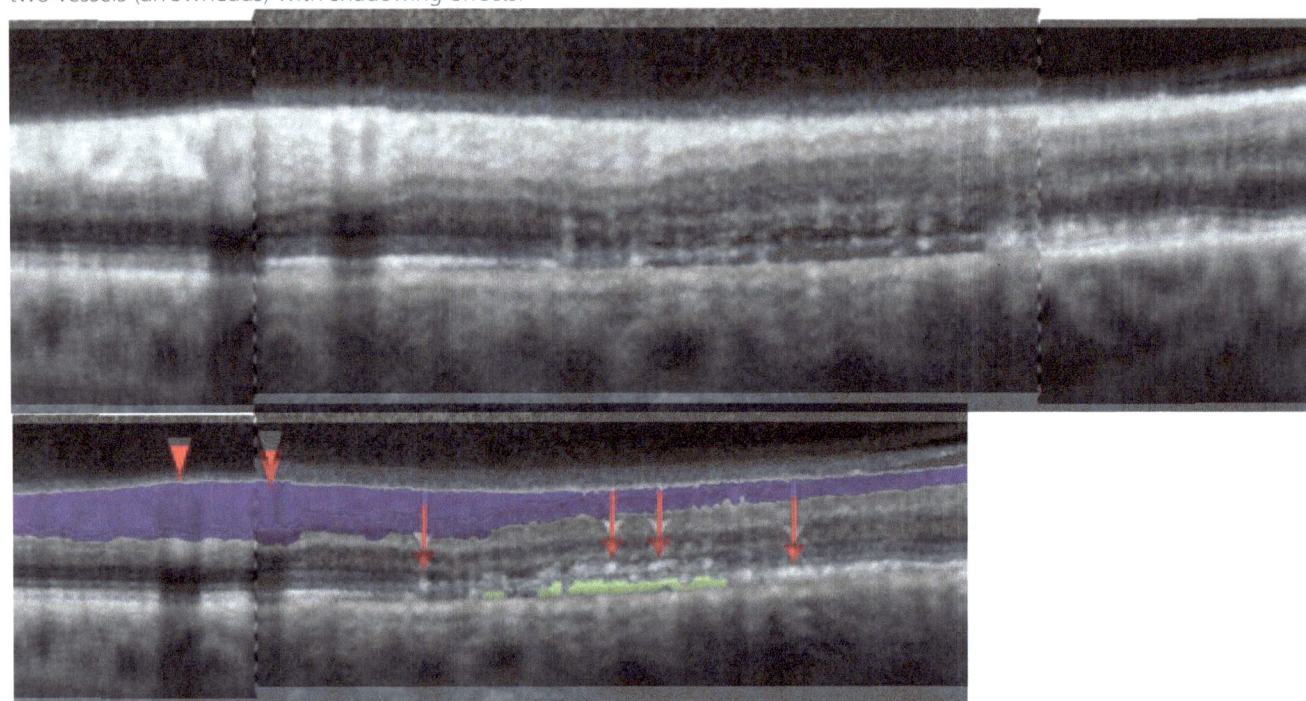

The patient below also has subretinal fluid (shaded red) from active central serous chorioretinopathy. Notice the subtle presence of a PED (shaded orange) between the RPE (shaded green) and Bruch's membrane (shaded yellow).

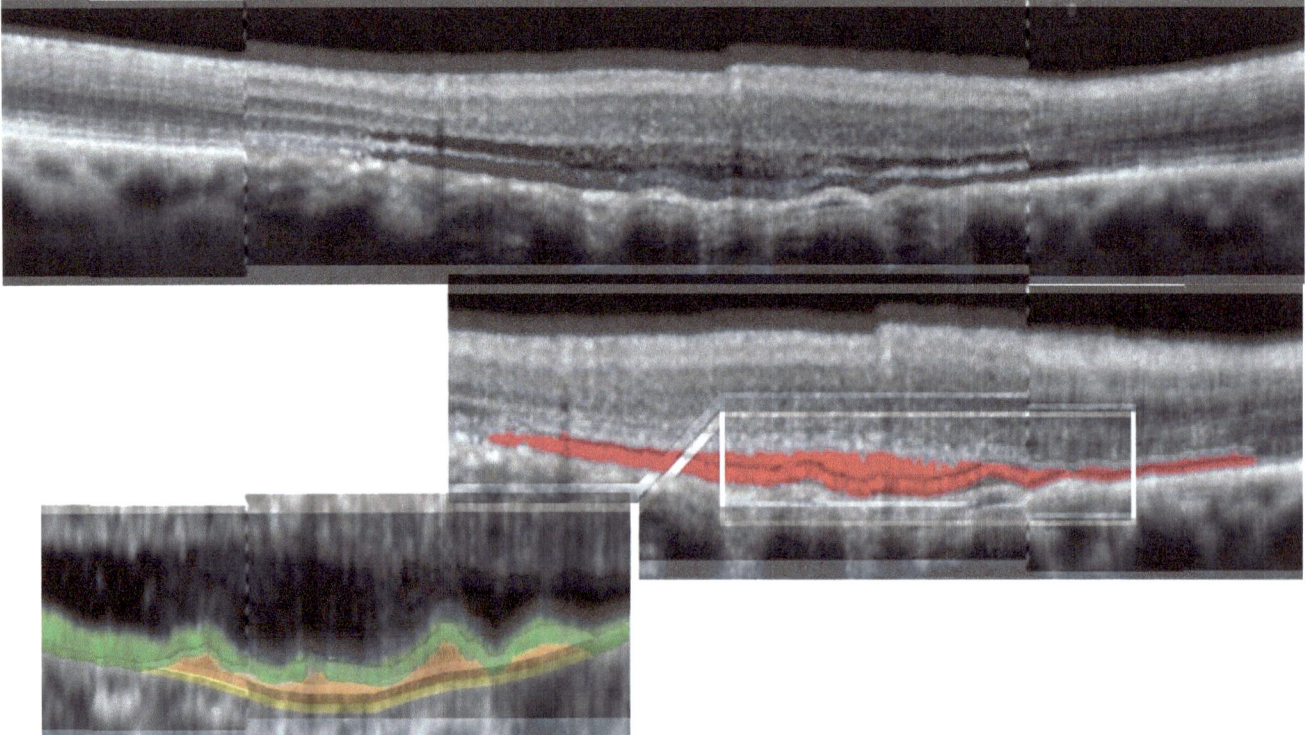

Multiple Pathologies

Multiple pathologic processes can occur within the same patient. It is important to examine the OCT carefully to rule out or rule in concurrent pathologies. In the OCT image below, the patient has a full thickness macular hole with intraretinal cysts predominantly in the outer nuclear layer but also within the inner nuclear layer. On close inspection of the RPE at the macular hole, small drusenoid PEDs are visible at the sides and center of the base of the hole.

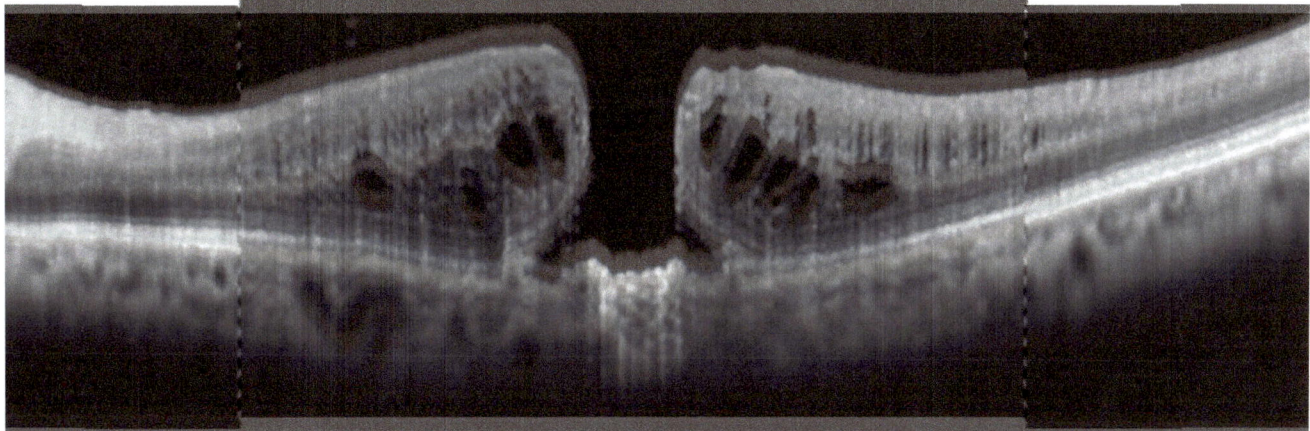

The OCT below is of the same patient as above, but through a slice tangential to the macular hole rather than through the center of the hole. Clinical examination discloses readily apparent drusen (arrow on left) that correspond to the drusenoid PEDs on the OCT (arrow on right). The arrows point to the exact same location on the fundus image and the OCT image:

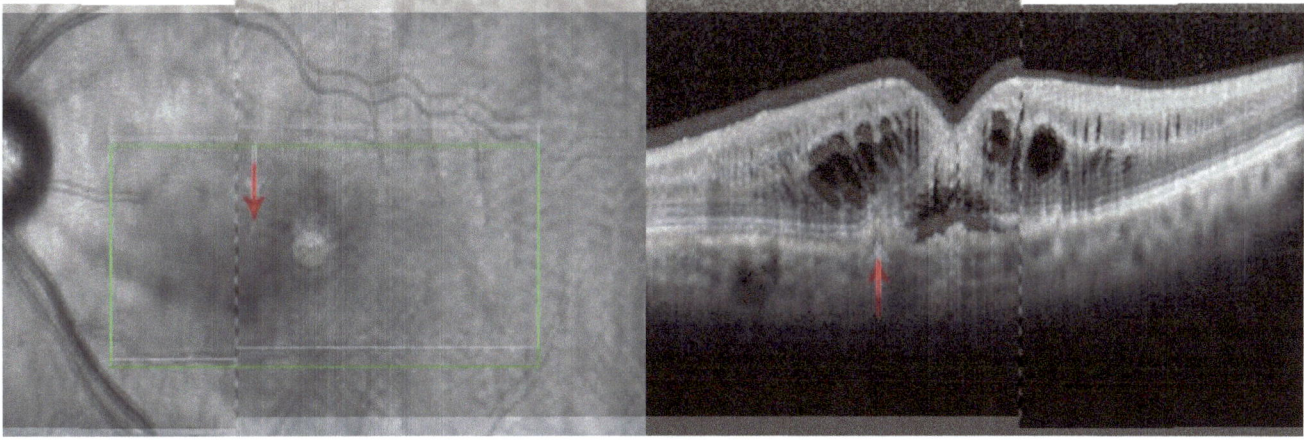

The patient below presents with an ERM, dry AMD, and multiple drusenoid PEDs. The "debris" is below the level of the RPE and there isn't any choroidal neovascularization or leakage observable on fluorescein or high-speed ICG angiography. Notice that overlying the largest of the drusenoid PEDs, the photoreceptor outer nuclear layer is visibly thinned (arrow):

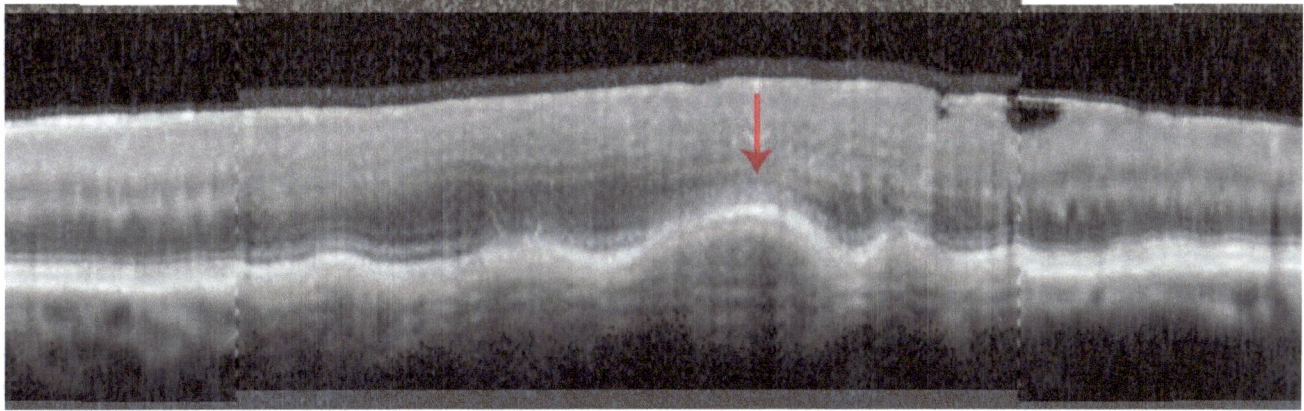

Multiple Pathologies

In the OCT image below, multiple drusenoid PEDs are visible in this patient with dry AMD. Choroidal neovascularization is not visible with contact lens biomicroscopy nor with fluorescein or ICG angiography. The drusenoid material is located below the level of the RPE. The ellipsoid zone of the photoreceptors appears slightly less bright and crisp in some areas overlying the drusenoid PEDs. The patient also has a lamellar macular hole. Notice that the inner nuclear layer abruptly ends at this lamellar hole.

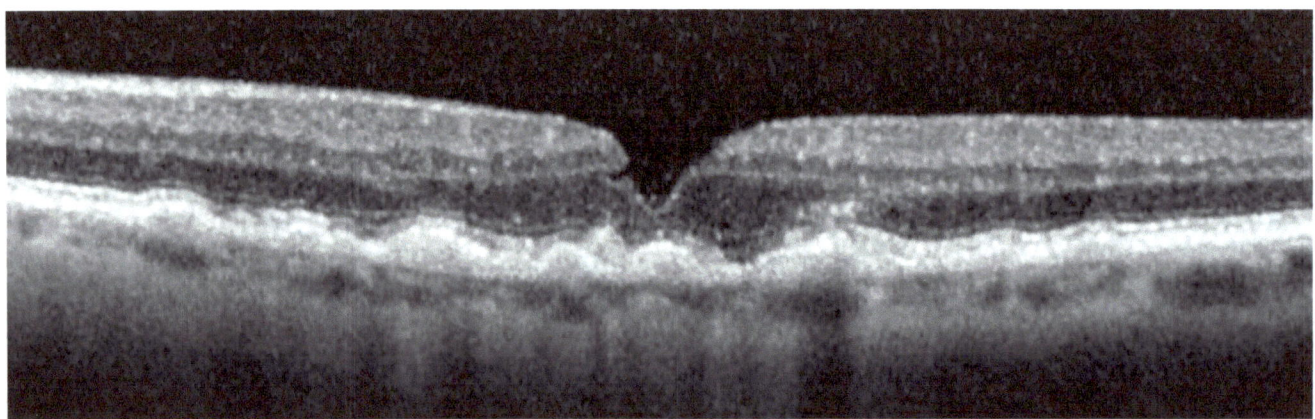

The image below was taken from a diabetic patient who presents with dry AMD and non-proliferative diabetic retinopathy. Slit lamp fundoscopy confirmed numerous hard exudates as well as retinal thickening located temporal to the fovea. The OCT shows the presence of hard exudates within multiple layers of the retina and retinal thickening in the vicinity of the hard exudates. The patient also has posterior vitreous floaters near the fovea.

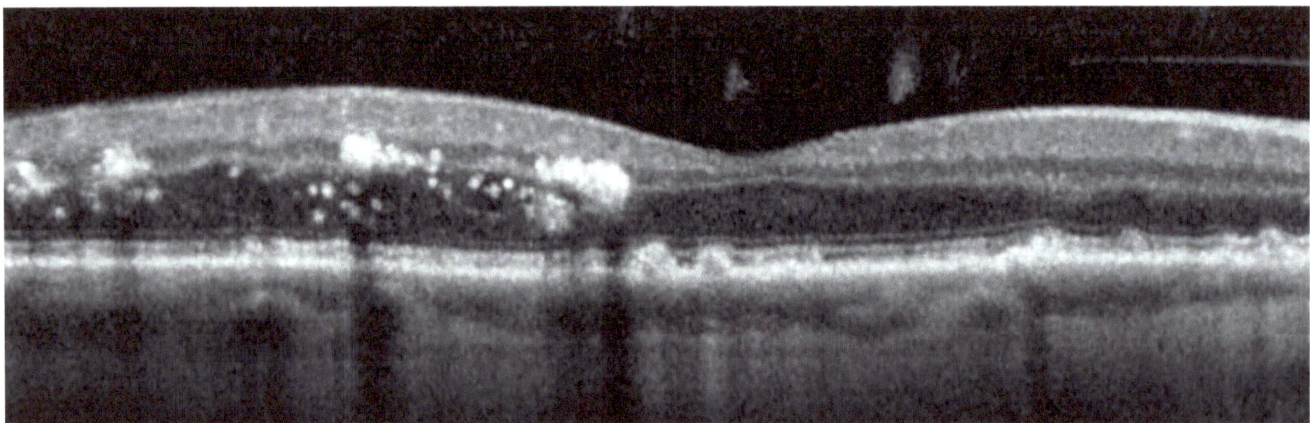

About the Author

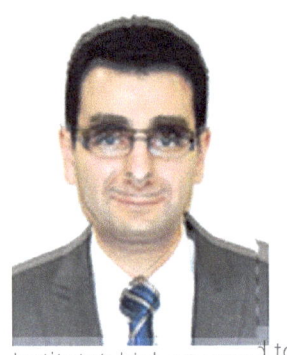

NEAL A. ADAMS, M.D. is a consulting vitreo-retinal physician and surgeon in the greater Washington D.C. area.

He is the former Chairman of the Department of Ophthalmology at the Paul L. Foster School of Medicine at the Texas Tech University Health Sciences Center. Prior to his position in Texas, he was Chief of the Division of Visual Physiology at the Wilmer Eye Institute of the Johns Hopkins Hospital, Johns Hopkins University School of Medicine.

Dr. Adams earned his bachelors in chemistry from Yale University and his M.D. from Johns Hopkins University School of Medicine. He is a graduate of the Johns Hopkins Hospital's Wilmer Eye Institute Residency Program. Following completion of a Retina Fellowship at Wilmer, he was selected to join the Faculty at Johns Hopkins and honored with Johns Hopkins Wilmer Eye Institute's highest award to a junior faculty member: the Maumenee Scholar. He was then selected as Chief of the Division of Visual Physiology. Dr. Adams is Board-Certified in ophthalmology.

Dr. Adams devotes time to research on retinal disorders and has coined a new category of retinal degenerations called the "retinal ciliopathies."

He is currently Editor in Chief of the peer-reviewed ophthalmic medical journal *Eye Reports*. Dr. Adams has authored numerous publications, including the book *Nutrition for the Eye*. He has appeared on ABC, CBS, and Fox News programs. His expert analysis has appeared in papers across the country, including *The Washington Post*, *The New York Times*, and *The Boston Globe*, as well as in a *US News & World Report's Good Vision Guide*.

www.ingramcontent.com/pod-product-compliance
Lightning Source LLC
Chambersburg PA
CBHW051934210526
45473CB00006B/2247